S0-ABD-040

Do I have to wear garlic around my neck?

Family remedies for holistic healing.

by Adrienne Selko

 **Interex • USA**

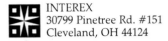 INTEREX
30799 Pinetree Rd. #151
Cleveland, OH 44124

CIP 96-94390
ISBN 0-9653220-0-9

Design Randy Martin

Cover illustration Ethan Gould
Dedication page illustration Tori Gould
Back cover photograph William Gould

Manufactured in the United States of America
10 9 8 7 6 5 4 3 2 1

All material in this publication is provided for information only and may not be construed as medical advice or instruction. No action or inaction should be taken solely on the contents of this publication: instead, readers should consult appropriate health professionals on any matter relating to their health and well-being. The information and opinions provided in this publication are believed to be accurate and sound, based on the best judgment available to the author, and readers who fail to consult with appropriate health authorities assume the risk of any injuries.

Dedication

To my husband,
    my soulmate   *- Philip Gould*

To my children,
    my heart   *- Ethan & Tori*

To my parents,
    my everlasting source of inspiration
        - Shirley & Phillip Selko

To my sister,
    my best friend   *- Allison Selko*

To my brother in law,
    my comrade-in-arms   *- David Brownstein*

To my nieces,
    the future   *- Hailey & Jessica*

To my grandmother,
    my model of character and strength
        - Esther Zapiler

To my grandfather,
    who I always feel smiling down on me from above
        - Papa Lou z"l

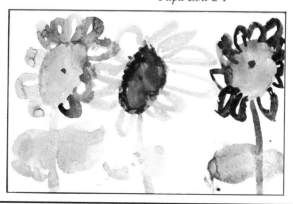

Acknowledgments

Special thanks to Jay Seaton, my mentor and friend, for supporting my vision for many years.

My appreciation to Randy Martin the designer of this book. His creativity and wisdom helped bring this book to fruition.

Thanks to Susan Martin for editing and proofing.

Thanks to family and friends who encouraged me to write this book.

And to my friend, Emily Hoffman, whose response upon hearing that I was writing a book on family remedies for holistic healing was:

"Do I have to wear garlic around my neck?"

Forward

I am excited to be involved with "Do I Have to Wear Garlic Around My Neck: Family Remedies for Holistic Healing" because I believe these remedies are safe and effective. I frequently employ many of these vitamin and herb recommendations for use in my practice.

People around the world are familiar with the medicinal benefits of natural substances (such as herbs, vitamins, etc.). I feel very strongly that these substances are undervalued in western medicine. Natural substances are useful by themselves as well as in combination with traditional medical therapy when indicated.

This book provides a simple, easy-to-use guide to many common ailments. What I find particularly useful is the food source reference for each condition. I cannot say enough about how much a healthy diet means for improving one's overall health.

I am pleased to recommend this book as a safe and natural way to treat many common ailments.

David A. Brownstein, M.D.

David A. Brownstein

Why did I write this book?

My story is simple.

Four years ago my son had an acute case of bronchitis. I rushed him to the pediatrician's office where they threw a mask over his face, attached a tube to a machine, and gave me steroid pills for him to take. My son was a real trooper but I just sat in the chair and cried.

That day I told myself there had to be a better way. I hit the library, spoke to everyone I knew and came up with a holistic approach to treat his bouts of bronchitis. For four years now I have treated him and my daughter holistically. We have practically eliminated the need for antibiotics. Doctor's visits are for illnesses that can only be cured with medical intervention.

Along the way I picked up a lot of knowledge about ways to treat a variety of common ailments. This is what I offer to you.

The philosophy I have worked so hard to formulate predates my existence by thousands of years. I have uncovered what my ancestors have always known. Balance is the key to good health. Your body, mind and spirit must be in balance.

Illness is the body's way of getting your attention. Something is off balance. Amazingly, we possess the ability to regain our balance. Utilizing the abundance of resources that nature offers us, we can recover our health.

Experience has taught me that the combination of herbs, vitamins, food sources and home remedies is the most effective and efficient method to treat our most common ailments.

Have you ever sat down to read a book about remedies for common ailments and found that you didn't know enough to even read the book because it was so complicated? You had to read about the origin of the plant, the climate of the country and the various methods of preparation. All of this before you could even use the one piece of information that might help you!

This book will make it easy for you.

Simplicity is the key. The teas, vitamins and foods are all within reach. You do not need to travel to Outer Mongolia to cure your tension headache, although a trip away from home might just be the cure.

Only 35 herbs are used in this book. These herbs were chosen based on their positive results and the ease of acquiring them. All are available at either grocery or health food stores.

The vitamin section can be used in a variety of ways. You can take vitamins in tablet form or you can choose either food or herbal sources as a method to obtain vitamins.

Most importantly the home remedies will be easy to perform and I will guide you through them.

No search and find missions are necessary to use this book. All information that pertains to each ailment will be included in the chapter that discusses that ailment.

I do understand your heartfelt thanks.

Adrienne Selko

How to use this book

Like the information presented on these pages, this book is easy to use. It is divided into 5 sections.

Section 1 *VITAMINS*
Vitamins can be taken
in a variety of ways.

The most beneficial way of bringing vitamins into your diet is through food or herbal sources. For each vitamin there will be a list of food sources and herbal sources. Generally speaking, steam or stir-fry vegetables to prevent loss of vitamins while cooking.

In some cases, you cannot get a large enough concentration of a particular vitamin simply through food. Because you would have to consume such vast quantities of food that it would lead to other ailments listed in this book, you should use a vitamin supplement which is available at grocery stores, drug stores, discount stores or health food stores.

Section 2 *HERBS*
Herbs can be used as teas, foods
or healing agents.

Herbs are found both in individual teas or in combination teas. Hot liquids and steam from the tea have their own healing properties. Sometimes a tincture made from the herb is the most effective method to utilize medicinal properties. Herbal baths or compresses are often very effective in treating certain ailments. You can also add herbs to your diet.

Section 3 FOOD
Foods to eat andfoods to avoid.

Here you will find a list of foods which are particularly good to eat when you have a specific ailment. There is also a list of foods to avoid.

Section 4 HOME REMEDIES
Home remedies that are easy to do.

Many home remedies you have heard from your grandmother. Others seem to make sense intuitively once you consider them. In some cases, the fact that you are helping yourself get better contributes to the cure. Instructions, and dosages when necessary, will be included. Of the many effective home remedies, I chose those which take a short period of time to prepare and use.

Section 5 A FEW MORE IDEAS
Additional information.

This section applies in some cases when I just had to pass along information even if it didn't fit neatly into a category. How can I sleep at night if I haven't passed along all of my useful knowledge?

Warning:

Herbs, vitamins and food are powerful healers!

The power of nature must be respected. Take the time to learn your own body. Consult a qualified knowledgeable person who can help you decide which herbs and vitamins work best with your system. Dosages are very important, just as they would be for any healing agent or man-made drug.

Throughout this book I will indicate which herbs should be used with caution. Some herbs cannot be taken during pregnancy. Some herbs cannot be taken if you have other conditions such as high blood pressure, heart disease, diabetes, etc.

Included in this book is a table of herbs about which the experts disagree. Some consider these herbs dangerous, others will use with caution. Generally I do not include these herbs in this book, however don't rule them out entirely when discussing your course of treatment with a professional health expert.

Table of Contents

Chapter

1

ALLERGIES

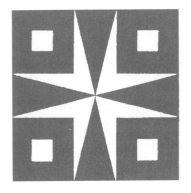

The modern day version
of that bad apple that
Adam ate.
And mankind shall
suffer from allergies.

For many years, my sister and I watched my mother place her face over a cup of steaming tea. We sat in awe as our mother tried to reach a higher state of consciousness through meditation. It turns out she was merely inhaling the steam of the tea; a perfect remedy for allergies, coughs, colds, and congestion.

A discussion of allergies is absolutely incomplete without mentioning that the content of our processed food is often the culprit. Sulfites in food can even be fatal to some people. Laws now require sulfite to be listed in packaged foods. Check labels carefully as sometimes the word sulfite is part of another word. Many people are allergic to yellow dye, also known as tartrazine. There is yellow dye in practically everything, so watch out!

ALLERGIES

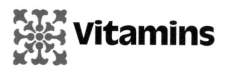 **Vitamins**

These are the vitamins that have been shown to help people suffering from allergies.

A	B12	E
B3	B Complex	F
B5	C	H
B6		

Food sources of Vitamins

Herb sources of vitamins

A
Carrots, dairy, fish liver oil, fruits (yellow), lemon grass, liver, milk, margarine, okra, vegetables (green, yellow).

A
Alfalfa, burdock, capsicum, dandelion, garlic, kelp, marsh-mallow, papaya, parsley, rasp-berry, red clover, safflower, watercress, yellow dock.

B3
Avocados, broccoli, carrots, corn flour, dates, eggs, figs, fish, liver, meat (lean), peanuts (roasted), potatoes, poultry (white meat), prunes, toma-toes, wheat germ, whole wheat, yeast.

B3
Alfalfa, burdock dandelion, fenugreek, kelp, parsley sage.

B5
Beans, bran, chicken, eggs, fish (saltwater), kidney, liver, mo-lasses ,nuts, pork, potatoes,

ALLERGIES

Food sources of Vitamins	*Herb sources of vitamins*

tomatoes, vegetables (green), wheat germ, whole grains.

B6
Bananas, cantaloupe, eggs, kidney, liver, milk, nuts, soybeans, vegetables (green leafy), wheat bran, wheat germ.

B6
Alfalfa.

B12
Beef, cheese, clams, eggs, fish, kidney, lamb, liver, milk, oysters, sardines, tofu.

B12
Alfalfa, kelp.

B Complex
Apples, bananas, beans, beets, cabbage, carrots, cauliflower, corn, grapefruit, liver, mushrooms, onions, oranges, peas, peanuts, potatoes, spinach, turnips, watercress, yeast.

C
Berries, black currants, broccoli, brussels sprouts, cabbage, cantaloupe, cauliflower, cherry juice (acerola), citrus fruits, guava, horseradish, kiwi, peppers (red, green), potatoes, rose hips, spinach, strawberries, tomatoes, turnips, vegetables (green leafy), watercress.

C
Alfalfa, burdock, boneset, catnip, capsicum, chickweed, dandelion, garlic, hawthorn, horseradish, kelp, parsley, plantain, papaya, rose hips, shepherd's purse, strawberry, watercress, yellow dock.

ALLERGIES

Food sources of Vitamins	Herb sources of vitamins
E Broccoli, brown rice, cereals (whole grain), corn, eggs, kidnesy, liver, peas, spinach, sweet potatoes, vegetables (green leafy), vegetable oils, wheat germ.	**E** Alfalfa, dandelion, gotu kola, kelp.

F
Almonds, avocados, black currant oil, cod liver oil, corn oil, cottonseed oil, flaxseed oil, primrose oil, sunflower oil, safflower oil, soybean oil, linseed oil, peanuts, pecans, wheat germ.

H
Bran, brewer's yeast, chicken, egg yolks, fish (saltwater), fruits, lamb, liver, kidney, milk, molasses, nuts, rice (unrefined), pork, sprouts, wheat germ, vegetables (green leafy), yogurt.

ALLERGIES
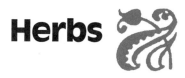

Herbs

These are the herbs that have been shown to help people suffering from allergies.

Stinging Nettles -
   (freeze dried)
Echinacea
Elder
Bayberry
Ephedra*

Burdock
Dandelion
Pleurisy root
Red clover
Blessed thistle

*When used properly, this drug is perfectly safe.

Food

These are the foods that have been shown to help people suffering from allergies.

Hot chili peppers
Hot curry
Garlic
Raw seeds and nuts
Fruits

Vegetables
Grains
Orange juice
Horseradish
Raw honey

These are the foods that have been shown to aggravate or cause allergies.*

Wheat
Eggs
Dairy products
Caffeine

Chocolate
Shellfish
Strawberries
Tomatoes

Citrus
Red meat
Hot spices

*Systematically eliminate these foods from your diet to determine your particular culprits.

ALLERGIES

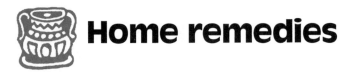 **Home remedies**

SWEET SOLUTION
*   Bee Pollen. Take two teaspoons daily. (It's also available in capsules.)

A YOGURT A DAY ...
*   Eat yogurt daily for three months *before* the allergy season. This can lessen the suffering during allergy season.

A SPOT OF TEA
*   Drink stinging nettle tea daily November-April. Drink fenugreek tea a month prior to the allergy season.

FOOD ALLERGY DRINK
*   To a glass of water add the ever popular apple cider vinegar and honey. Sip with meals. Relieves allergic reaction to food.

DAILY REMINDER
*   Daily doses of garlic and horseradish build up resistance.

HAY FEVER HOP
*   Vigorous exercise such as skipping rope or even riding a stationary bike helps. Part of the assistance comes from a constricting effect of small blood vessels. In some cases this can soothe hay fever symptoms in less than 5 minutes.

ALLERGIES
Home remedies

CATCH THAT NOSE

* For a runny nose you can dry a 1-inch square of tangerine peel. Leave it at room temperature for one week. Then store in an airtight container. Chew and swallow one square to dry up a drippy nose.

COMBO PLATE

* To strengthen your cell walls and build immunity, blend together brewer's yeast, grapefruit and wheat germ. Drink up.

PITCH A TENT IN YOUR KITCHEN

* This healing tent is a steam tent. Using any of the following oils: eucalyptus, thyme, rosemary, lavender. Add 5-6 drops to 2 or 3 cups of boiling water. Place a towel over your head and over the bowl containing the drops of oil, thus forming a tent. Stay in your tent for 10 minutes. Use these 10 minutes to solve the issue of world peace.

ALLERGIES

 # A few more ideas

The most common food allergies are to tomatoes, citrus fruit, cow's milk, peanuts, chocolate, wheat products and peas.

The symptoms of allergies can cause other ailments. For example, an allergic reaction to food, such as a dripping nose, could end up as bronchitis. Therefore, with any constantly reoccuring condition, don't forget to check for allergies.

Chapter

2

ASTHMA

Inhale nature's
remedies,
exhale freely.

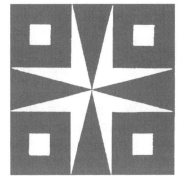

At the start of an asthma attack, my cousin Marc immediately grabs the newspaper and runs to the bathroom. Turning on the shower, to hot of course, he lets the steam fill the bathroom. Sitting in the steam for 15-20 minutes allows his airways to open up. An added benefit is that he learns which senators were indicted that week.

I include asthma in this book because so many people suffer from it and the numbers are increasing. Because asthma is serious and sometimes can be fatal, you must be under the care of a health professional.

The following are measures you can take to assist in treating the condition. You must let your health professional know which vitamins and especially which herbs you want to use. Do not do this on your own!

ASTHMA

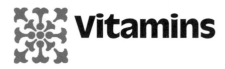 **Vitamins**

These are the vitamins that have been shown to help people suffering from asthma.

A	Choline	D	P
B6	Folic Acid	E	
B12	Inositol	F	
B15	C	H	

Food sources of Vitamins

A
Carrots, dairy products, fish liver oil, fruits (yellow), lemon grass, liver, milk, margarine, okra, vegetables (green and yellow).

B6
Avocado, bananas, brewer's yeast, cantaloupe, chicken, eggs, liver, kidney, milk, nuts, oats, peanuts, peas, potatoes, soybeans, vegetables (green leafy), walnuts, wheat bran, wheat germ.

B12
Carrots, potatoes, turnips, whey (liquid from curdled milk), yogurt.

Herb sources of Vitamins

A
Alfalfa, burdock, capsicum, dandelion, garlic, kelp, marshmallow, papaya, parsley, raspberry, red clover, safflower, watercress, yellow dock.

B6
Alfalfa.

B12
Alfalfa, kelp.

ASTHMA

Food sources of Vitamins

Herb sources of Vitamins

B15
Apricot kernels, brewer's yeast, brown rice (whole), pumpkin seeds, sesame seeds, whole grains.

B Factor: Choline
Egg yolk, brain, brewer's yeast, fish, heart, liver, peas, peanut butter, seeds, soybeans, turnips, vegetables (green leafy), wheat germ.

B Factor: Folic Acid
Apricots, asparagus, avocados, beans, broccoli, carrots, cantaloupe, chick peas, egg yolks, flour (dark rye, whole, wheat), liver, mushrooms, oranges, pumpkin, soybeans, spinach, sprouts, vegetables (green leafy), yeast (tourtula), yogurt.

B Factor: Inositol
Brains, brewer's yeast, cabbage, cantaloupe, grapefruit, heart, lima beans (dried), liver, molasses, oatmeal, oranges, peanuts, raisins, sesame seeds, soybeans, wheat germ, whole wheat bread.

ASTHMA

Food sources of Vitamins	Herb sources of Vitamins

C

Berries, black currants, broccoli, brussels sprouts, cabbage, cantaloupe, cauliflower, cherry juice (acerola), citrus fruits, guava, horseradish, kiwi, peppers (red, green), potatoes, rose hips, spinach, strawberries, tomatoes, turnips, vegetables (green leafy), watercress.

C

Alfalfa, burdock, boneset, catnip, capsicum, chickweed, dandelion, garlic, hawthorn, horseradish, kelp, parsley, plantain, papaya, rose hips, shepherd's purse, strawberry, watercress, yellow dock.

D

Dairy, egg yolks, fish liver oils, herring, milk, salmon, spinach, tuna.

D

Alfalfa, watercress.

E

Broccoli, brown rice, brussels sprouts, cereals (whole grains), corn, eggs, flour (enriched), liver, nuts, peas, soybeans, sweet potatotes, spinach, vegetables (green leafy), vegetable oils, wheat germ, whole wheat.

E

Alfalfa, dandelion, gotu kola, kelp, raspberry, rose hips, watercress.

F

Almonds, avocados, black currant oil, cod liver oil, corn oil, cottonseed oil, flaxseed oil, linseed oil, peanuts, pecans, primrose, sunflower, safflower oils, soybean oil, wheat germ.

ASTHMA

Food sources of Vitamins

Herb sources of Vitamins

H

Beef, bran, brewer's yeast, chicken, egg yolks, fish (salt-water), fruit, lamb, liver, kidney, milk, molasses, nuts, rice (unrefined), pork, sprouts, soy flour, wheat germ, vegetables (green leafy).

P

Apricots, blackberries, black currants, buckwheat, cherries, citrus fruits (white skin and segment membranes), grapes, peppers (green), plums, prunes, rose hips, spinach.

Herbs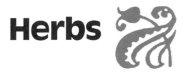

These are the herbs that have been shown to help people suffering from asthma.

Mullein	Echinacea	Ginkgo - An extract from
Thyme	Horsetail	the ginkgo leaf is the
Lemon thyme	Slippery elm	number one prescription
Black cohost	Ephedra*	for asthma in Germany.
Fenugreek		

* When used properly, this herb is perfectly safe.

ASTHMA

 Food

These are the foods that have been shown to help people suffering from asthma.

Apples	Hot chili peppers	Shellfish:
Apricots	Black beans	crab
Ginger	Green beans	clams
Garlic	Onions	mussels
Vegetables	Peaches	oysters
Nuts	Turnips	Cabbage
Seeds	Horseradish	Carrots
Oatmeal	Salmon	Celery
Brown rice	Sardines	Cherries
Whole grains	Haddock	Tabasco sauce
Fish oil	Mackerel	

Coffee - I don't usually recommend this but in the case of asthma some people have found that strong coffee can ease an attack.

These are the foods that have been shown to aggravate asthma.

Cold beverages	Fish	Nuts
Alfalfa	Red meat	Eggs
Beets	Pork	White flour
Carrots	Salt	White sugar
Dairy products	Spinach	Cola
Corn oil	Turkey	Bananas
Safflower oil	Chicken	Tofu
Sunflower oil		

ASTHMA

Home remedies

TOXINS BE GONE
  * Mix distilled water with lemon juice. Drink 3 cups per day. This tasty drink can rid the body of toxins and mucus.

GO AHEAD, DRINK
  * Drink ½ to 1 cup of fluid per hour at room temperature or warmer. This keeps mucus thin and coughable. Sorry for the gory details.

QUICK, GRAB THIS
  * At the onset of an attack drink any of the following: hot apple cider, hot lemonade, herbal tea. This may stop an attack cold.

WHEEZE BE GONE
  * Add 1 teaspoon of apple cider vinegar to a glass of water. Sip for ½ hour. Wait 30 minutes and then repeat. For nighttime wheezing try drinking 1 teaspoon of either corn oil or sunflower oil before bedtime.

NOT FOR THE FAINT OF HEART
  * Eat one or more raw minced garlic cloves. Do not give this to children. In the 1800's a favorite cure for asthma was a concoction of garlic cloves boiled with vinegar and sugar taken by the spoonful each morning.

FAVORITE OF THE CZAR
  * An old Russian folk remedy--inhale the steam of a boiling potato.

ASTHMA
Home remedies

STOP & WRAP
- ✶ At the first sign of wheezing saturate a couple of pieces of white cloth in white vinegar. Wrap around wrists. Sometimes it can stop a full-blown attack.

A NEW DRINK MENU
- ✶ Wild Cherry Bark Tea - Drink one cup before each meal and a cup at bedtime.
- ✶ Fresh Carrot Juice.
- ✶ Ginger Juice - Grate fresh ginger. Strain through a cheese-cloth and drink the remaining juice.

THE BREATHING BERRY
- ✶ Cranberries are believed to contain an ingredient that dilates the bronchial tubes and helps restore normal breathing. The best method of preparation is to cook, mash, and store cranberries in a glass jar. Keep this in the refrigerator. When an attack occurs mix 2 teaspoons of cranberries in hot water and sip.

BREATH OF FRESH AIR
- ✶ Yoga and other breathing methods can teach someone with asthma how to improve their breath capacity. (There are also types of massages and bodywork that can help.)

A LITTLE NIGHTCAP?
- ✶ On a plate next to your bed place thin slices of raw onion on a plate. Spread with honey and let it sit there overnight. Take 1 teaspoon of the remaining liquid, 4 times daily. This is also used as a contraceptive. (Just kidding, but it is hardly the seductive aroma of romance.)

ASTHMA
Home remedies

WHAT'S OLD IS NEW AGAIN

✱ Remember the stories of castor oil? Well, for asthma a castor oil pack on the back around the lung and kidney area helps. To make, place oil in a pan. Heat, but do not boil. Apply to area. Cover with plastic and then cotton. Put heating pad over the cotton and use ½ hour to an hour as needed.

THE OLD STANDBY

✱ Chicken Soup to the rescue. (See Colds for details on chicken soup.) In the case of asthma, chicken soup helps stop the migration of white blood cells to the respiratory passages. The more white blood cells, the more the area becomes inflamed.

ASTHMA

 A few more ideas

A brand new study out of Johns Hopkins found a link between food allergy and asthma in children. Allergic foods such as eggs, wheat, cow's milk, soy and fish were tested. If a child with asthma ingests one of these allergic foods, it could trigger an attack.

Also, children with a history of skin rash or skin allergies should be tested for asthma.

Chapter

3

BRONCHITIS

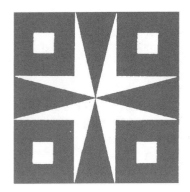

The cough
heard 'round
the world.
It jump started
our journey
into
holistic
healing!

C an you feel fondly about an illness? Had it not been for my son's bronchitis, my family would not be enjoying our holistic, healthy approach to medical care.

Some children wake up in the morning, grab a bowl of cereal and watch TV until school. Not my son. Not if he has a cough. Upon waking he soaks his feet in a mustard powder solution, while balancing a cup of herbal tea. Sitting on a table in front of him is the lovely morning combination of cereal and chicken soup. Separate bowls! His morning juice has Vitamin C crystals in it, of course. If the cough is severe he'll get a mustard plaster on his chest, and his last course is a Vitamin B12 shot in the tush. He does manage to watch TV throughout this routine. Then it's off to school.

BRONCHITIS

 Vitamins

These are the vitamins that have been shown to help people suffering from bronchitis.

A
B6
B12

C - Double your daily intake. If that proves to be too much the only symptom will be diarrhea. Reduce your amount but still keep taking it.

Food sources of Vitamins

A
Carrots, dairy, fish liver oil, fruit (yellow), lemon grass, liver, milk, margarine, okra, vegetables (green and yellow).

B6
Avocados, bananas, brewer's yeast, cantaloupe, chicken, eggs, kidney, liver, milk, nuts, oats peanuts, peas, potatoes, soybeans, vegetables (green leafy), walnuts, wheat bran, wheat germ.

B12
Beef, cheese, clams, cottage cheese, eggs, fish, lamb, liver, kidney, milk, oysters, sardines, tofu.

Herb sources of Vitamins

A
Alfalfa, burdock, capsicum, dandelion, garlic, kelp, marshmallow, papaya, parsley, raspberries, red clover, safflower, watercress, yellow dock.

B6
Alfalfa.

B12
Alfalfa, kelp.

BRONCHITIS

Food sources of Vitamins

C

Berries, black currants, broccoli, brussels sprouts, cabbage, cantaloupe, cauliflower, cherry juice (acerola), citrus fruits, guava, horseradish, kiwi, peppers (red and green), potatoes, rose hips, spinach, strawberries, tomatoes, turnips, watercress, vegetables (green leafy).

Herb sources of Vitamins

C

Alfalfa, burdock, boneset, catnip, capsicum, chickweed, dandelion, garlic, hawthorn, horseradish, kelp, parsley, plantain, papaya, rose hips, shepherd's purse, strawberry, watercress, yellow dock.

Herbs

These are the herbs that have been shown to help people suffering from bronchitis.

Elecampane	Horehound	Yarrow	Yellow dock
Pleurisy root	Lungwort	Thyme	Peppermint
Ma Huang	Slippery elm	Anise	Goldenseal
Ephedra*	Ginseng	Wild cherry	Fenugreek

*When used properly, this drug is perfectly safe.

Foods

These are the foods that have been shown to help people suffering from bronchitis.

Garlic	Onions	Chicken soup	Black pepper
Bell pepper	Mustard	Black beans	Honey
Oranges	Curry (spice)	Salsa (hot)	
Licorice	Fish oil	Horseradish	

BRONCHITIS

Foods

These are the foods have been shown to aggravate bronchitis.

Dairy products	Avocados
Bananas	Tofu

 Home remedies

SERGEANT, CATCH THAT COUGH

* The police suggest a hefty dose of chicken soup. Heavy garlic can chase off the perpetrator. Next take the victim's feet and place in a bowl of warm water to which 1 heaping tablespoon of mustard powder is added. Soak until it becomes uncomfortable. This draws the offending germs out of the chest and to the feet. Arresting the cough and symptoms is the best way to reduce this crime.

TAKE COVER

* Cover the chest with a mustard plaster. Make a paste out of mustard powder by using 2 tablespoons of flour, 1 tablespoon of mustard and some water. First place oil on the chest and then place the paste. Only let it sit for a little while as it really heats up. Again, you are drawing out the congestion.

RUB IT OUT

* Other chest rubs include Vics rubs or eucalyptus oil. At bedtime apply rub or oil and place flannel on top. It can work throughout the night.

BRONCHITIS
Home remedies

* Use essential oils but be careful because they are quickly absorbed by the skin. Mix with other oils. Also place a few drops of the oil on the bedsheets or pillow, the vapors will help.

* A unique chest rub. Take finely cut fresh onions that were fried in lard and apply to chest. Cover with a cloth and keep body warm with hot water bottles or a heating pad.

PROVISIONS

* Drink water every time you cough. This loosens the mucus.

* Herbal teas that contain Ma Huang, ephedra, horehound or pleurisy root are excellent. Any of the herbs listed above make great teas.

* Stir two tablespoons of raw honey in hot water and sip. Or combine honey with an equal amount of lemon juice and take by the spoonful as needed.

* Or honey with a kick--freshly grated horseradish combined with an equal part of honey taken daily with breakfast.

* A hearty spoonful of lemon juice and olive oil, in equal parts. A wonderful morning drink.

* A syrup of freshly cooked blackberry juice combined with equal amount of sugar. Tablespoon doses as needed.

BRONCHITIS
Home remedies

* Boil chopped figs in 2 cups of water for 6 minutes. Cover until cool and store in fridge. Sip 1/2 cup morning and evening.

HIT THE SHOWER
* A hot shower or a room steamed from a hot shower opens up the airways quickly. Steam from tea can be inhaled also. Place a towel over your head and form a tent.

SHOOT THE GERM
* A shot of vitamin B-12 works, especially for children. If given early it can sometimes prevent a full-blown case of bronchitis. Twice a day for one or two days should do it. Check with a qualified professional.

 A few more ideas

Bronchitis is a common ailment that sometimes starts as a cough and then leads to heavy breathing and can exhibit the same signs as asthma. Oftentimes allergies turn into bronchitis. The trick is to catch this cough before it turns into wheezing.

Chapter

4

COLDS/FLU

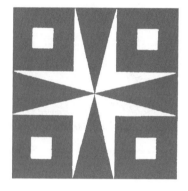

This ailment is
treasured for the
priceless advice
every relative feels
obligated to give you.

Smile politely,
but listen.
Their advice may be right.

For as long as I can remember, everyone in my family upon waking would eat little orange pills. These miracles pills were really Vitamin C tablets. Vitamin C is amazing for its ability to ward off colds. Sometimes this vitamin can outright prevent the cold; other times it will decrease the severity of the symptoms and shorten the length of the illness. Linus Pauling knew what he was talking about.

In every Jewish household there is one absolute truth---CHICKEN SOUP. Over 5,000 years of success has convinced us that it works for many ailments. Now there is scientific proof. A recent study at the University of California concluded that an amino acid called cysteine is present in chicken. Cysteine is chemically similar to acetylcysteine which is prescribed for respiratory infections. I was willing to take it on faith.

COLDS/FLU

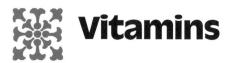 **Vitamins**

These are the vitamins that have been shown to help people suffering from colds/flu.

A	C
Beta-carotene	D
B Complex	P

Food sources of Vitamins

Herb sources of Vitamins

A
Carrots, dairy, fish liver oil, fruits (yellow), lemon grass, liver, milk, margarine, okra, vegetables (green, yellow).

A
Alfalfa, burdock, cayenne, dandelion, garlic, kelp, marshmallow, papaya, parsley, raspberry, red clover, safflower, watercress, yellow dock.

Beta-carotene
Carrots, apricots, cantaloupes, peaches, squash, sweet potato, tropical fruit, spinach, broccoli, collard greens, kale, peppers, pumpkins.

Beta-carotene
Bay leaves (crumbled), basil, marjoram, parsley, sage.

B Complex
Apples, bananas, beans, beets, cabbage, carrots, cauliflower, corn, grapefruit, kelp, mushrooms, onions, oranges, peas, peanuts, potatoes, spinach,

B Complex
Alfalfa, burdock, cayenne, dandelion, fenugreek, kelp, parsley, safflower, sage, watercress.

COLDS/FLU

Food sources of Vitamins

Herb sources of Vitamins

turnips, watercress.

C
Citrus fruits, currants, strawberries, cabbage, tomatoes, red pepper, kiwi, green pepper, broccoli, guava, brussels sprouts, turnips, spinach, watercress.

C
Alfalfa, burdock, boneset, catnip, cayenne, chickweed, dandelion, shepherd's purse, garlic, horseradish, kelp, parsley, plantain, papaya, rose hips, strawberries, yellow dock, watercress.

D
Milk, dairy products, egg yolk, tuna, sardines, herring, salmon, fish liver oils, spinach, ultraviolet sun rays.

D
Alfalfa, watercress.

P
Citrus fruits, apricots, blackberries, cherries, grapes, plums, rose hips, currants, prunes, spinach, green peppers, buckwheat.

P
Dandelion, rose hips.

COLDS/FLU

 # Herbs

These are the herbs that have been shown to help people suffering from colds/flu.

Echinacea[1]	Peppermint	Yarrow
Ginger	Elder	Forsythia[3]
Cayenne Pepper	Lemon balm	Boneset
Rose hips[2]	Lemon grass	Barley water[4]
Linden	Anise	Borage
Thyme	Fennel	Balm
Sage		

[1] 2 capsules every 4 hours at start of cold. [2] Usually found with Vitamin C in pill form. [3] especially for a stuffy nose. [4] for aches.

 # Food

These are the foods that have been shown to help people suffering from colds/flu.

Chicken soup	Lemon
Garlic	Yogurt
Onions	Shiitake mushrooms

These are the foods that have been shown to aggravate colds/flu.

Dairy products -
They increase the production of mucus.

COLDS/FLU

Home remedies

GINGER DRINK
* Grate fresh ginger into warm water. Steep 5-10 minutes. Before drinking add lemon, honey, cayenne pepper. Be careful with the cayenne.

SWEAT IT OUT
* Add a handful of ginger and cayenne capsules to a hot bath. This literally sweats out the toxins.

VISITORS BEWARE DRINK
* Combine garlic oil with an equal amount of water. Add onion juice. 1/2 teaspoon every hour will do the trick. Try not to exhale.

EASIER GARLIC DRINK
* To one cup boiling water add juice from 1 lemon, one minced garlic clove, and 1/8 - 1/2 teaspoon cayenne pepper. Sweeten with honey if necessary.

GRAPEFRUIT DRINK
* Cut two large unpeeled grapefruit into small pieces and simmer in one quart of water for 1/2 hour. Strain and add honey to taste. If possible drink the entire quart of liquid throughout the day.

JUICY TREAT
* Make a delicious drink from red beets and carrots. Don't forget to add those few drops of vegetable oil to make it taste just right. It works.

COLDS/FLU
Home remedies

NEW KIND OF BROTH
* ✱ Peel potatoes to 1/2 inch thick including the skin. Discard center of potato. Boil for 20-30 minute. Strain cool and drink.

REMEMBER TO INHALE
* ✱ Pour 5 drops of eucalyptus oil into a hot bath. Essential oils are easily absorbed through the skin.

NOT FOR THE FAINT OF HEART
* ✱ Place a piece of garlic in each side of the mouth between the teeth and cheek at the start of a cold.

COLD FEET
* ✱ Place a piece of ice on the bottom of the big toe. Repeat three times daily. This is a technique used by Oriental healers to activate the acupuncture point.

COOL IT
* ✱ Dip a towel in cold water and rub briskly over parts of the body.

UP YOUR NOSE
* ✱ Create a nasal spray with 1/4 teaspoon of vitamin C (power or crystals), garlic oil and salt in 1/2 cup of water. Squirt a little into each nostril.

COLDS/FLU
Home remedies

UP YOUR NOSE TWO
* An easier nasal technique is to inhale a little saltwater into each nostril at the beginning of a cold.

MASSAGE
* With a natural sponge or brush, dry massage over entire body. This stimulates circulation and brings blood to surface.

STEAM TENT
* Place 6 drops of eucalyptus oil in boiling water. Place towel over your head and inhale. Try to form a tent. This prevents the steam from escaping. Plus your family can't see you.

COLDS/FLU

 # A few more ideas

Here are a few more ideas that can help you deal with a cold.

Walking briskly outdoors in the winter helps you stay well.

Keep fresh air circulating through a sickroom.

Eat lightly so your body can focus all of its energy on fighting the cold.

Bars of soap are perfect places for germs to settle- use liquid antibacterial soap.

Incense can purify and disinfect. Try cinnamon, myrrh, sweet grass and sage.

Chapter

5

COLD SORES

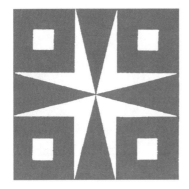

These are defined as
sores that turn up
at the wrong place
at the wrong time.
Enough said.

I t looks like grass. It's impossible to eat politely. And it always hangs out of a sandwich. This one crazy food is actually a wonder food and it's especially useful for cold sores.

What is it? It's ALFALFA. Alfalfa has more vitamins and minerals than most other foods and contains: Vitamins - A, B2 (Riboflavin), B3 (Niacin), B6, B12, C, D, E, G, K, T, U. Minerals-aluminum, calcium, chlorophyll, chlorine, fluorine, magnesium, phosphorus, potassium, selenium, silicon, sodium, sulfur, and trace minerals (boron, bromine, nickel, strontium, vanadium).

If the embarrassment of eating alfalfa overwhelms you, there ARE other options for treating cold sores. Read on.

COLD SORES

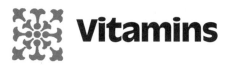 **Vitamins**

These are the vitamins that have been shown to help people suffering from cold sores.

A	C
Acidophilus*	E
B complex	

*This is found in supplement form or in active yogurt cultures.

Food sources of Vitamins

Herb sources of Vitamins

A
Carrots, dairy, fish liver oil, fruits (yellow), lemon grass, liver, milk, margarine, okra, vegetables (green leafy).

A
Alfalfa, burdock, capsicum, dandelion, garlic, kelp, marshmallow, papaya, parsley, raspberries, red clover, safflower, watercress, yellow dock.

B Complex
Apples, bananas, beans, beets, cabbage, carrots, cauliflower, corn, grapefruit, kelp, liver, mushrooms, onions, oranges, peas, peanuts, potatoes, spinach, turnips, watercress, yeast.

B Complex
Kelp.

C
Berries, black currants, broccoli, brussels sprouts, cabbage,

C
Alfalfa, burdock, boneset, catnip, capsicum, chickweed,

COLD SORES

Food sources of Vitamins

cantaloupe, cauliflower, cherry juice (acerola), citrus fruits, guava, horseradish, kiwi, peppers (red, green), potatoes, rose hips, spinach, strawberries, tomatoes, turnips, watercress, vegetables (green leafy).

E
Broccoli, brown rice, brussels sprouts, cereal (whole grain), corn, eggs, flour (enriched), liver, nuts, peas, soybeans, spinach, sweet potatoes, vegetables (green leafy), vegetable oils, wheat germ, whole wheat.

Herb sources of Vitamins

dandelion, garlic, hawthorn, horseradish, kelp, parsley, plantain, papaya, rose hips, shepherd's purse, strawberry, watercress, yellow dock.

E
Alfalfa, dandelion, gotu kola, kelp, raspberry, rose hips, watercress.

Herbs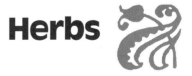

These are the herbs that have been shown to help people suffering from cold sores.

Lemon balm	Red clover
Goldenseal	Burdock
Echinacea	Yellow dock
Garlic	Dandelion

COLD SORES

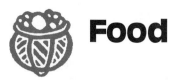 **Food**

These are the foods that have been shown to help people suffering from cold sores.

Alfalfa	Spinach	Sweet potatoes
Goat's milk	Eggs	Raw vegetables
Flax	Corn	Yogurt
Wheat germ	Liver	Garlic
Soybeans	Organ meats	Potatoes
Dulse	Brown rice	Sesame and all seeds
Watercress	Kelp	Green leafy vegetables
Broccoli		

These are the foods that have been shown to aggravate cold sores.

Peanuts	Nuts
Chocolate	Grains
Cola	Peas
Beer	Gelatin
Cereals	Chicken soup*

*It hurts me to write this.

COLD SORES

Home remedies

USE ON INSIDE AND OUTSIDE
* Drink buttermilk. Also apply it on the sore. The same for yogurt.

PUT IT ON ICE
* On a freshly erupted sore (that is about as delicately as I can put it) place a piece of ice. Keep it on about 40 minutes. It is said to bring healing within a day or two.

THE OUTER EDGE
* Find a pomegranate rind. Grind it up and boil 1 tablespoon worth in 1 ½ cups of water. Reduce mixture to 1 cup. Strain and apply to sore.

TEA TIME
* Into 1 cup of sage tea, add 1 teaspoon of powdered ginger. Drink several cups per day.

NEW & IMPROVED
* Use calendula ointment. Excellent healing properties.
* Combine 1 tablespoon of apple cider vinegar with 3 tablespoons of honey. Dab sore 3 times daily.
* Use a tincture* of myrrh or marigold.
* Cut a clove of garlic in half and rub on sore.
* Aloe Vera gel. Rub on sore. Works wonders.
* Vitamin E has healing properties. Open up a capsule and rub oil on sore.

*A tincture is a special method of preparing an herb.

COLDS SORES

 # A few more ideas

Cold sores originate with a form of the virus known as herpes simplex. Herpes appears in infancy and remains dormant until the body's defense mechanisms are weakened.

Factors that cause our bodies to weaken include: allergies, antibiotic medication, exhaustion, gastrointestinal problems, menstrual difficulties, sunburn, and stress.

We can treat the sores or they will go away of their own accord after a few weeks. However the virus always remains in our system.

Chapter
6
CHILDREN'S ISSUES

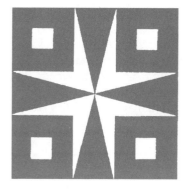

Give them a large
tablespoon of
self-confidence,
add a quart of love,
and mix it with a
positive attitude.
Voilà, you have
healthy children.

Prevention is the key. By starting early you can give children a diet which builds a strong immune system and allows them to fight off whatever is going around. Vitamins, herbs and home remedies are excellent to allow children to develop their own more powerful internal antibiotics.

Recent research has found that children are given so many antibiotics that certain diseases can become resistant. Used with caution, antibiotics work. But antibiotics work better with a strong, healthy immune system.

Because children are sensitive to certain foods for digestive or allergic reasons, this chapter does not include food and herbal sources for vitamins. Consult with a knowledgeable practitioner regarding the best method for your child to obtain vitamins.

CHILDREN'S ISSUES

Colds

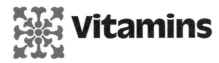 **Vitamins**

Vitamin C

Even as an infant, a child should take daily supplements of Vitamin C to build up the immune system and help prevent colds. When a child does get a cold, you can increase the dosage. Consult with a knowledgeable professional, however, because too much Vitamin C can cause diarrhea, which only aggravates a cold and can lead to dehydration in small children.(See "A few more ideas" on page 46.)

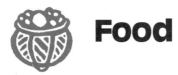 **Food**

These are the foods that have been shown to help children suffering from colds.

> Chicken soup[1]
> Fruits and vegetables
> Green vegetables[2]

[1]Chicken soup contains a natural antibiotic. See Chapter on Colds.
[2]Green vegetables, such as green pepper, broccoli, and green beans, open up the airways.

Just let the kids eat lightly. Most of their energy should go to fighting the cold and not to digesting food.

CHILDREN'S ISSUES
Colds
Food

These are the foods have been shown to aggravate colds in children.

Milk*   Bananas*
Cream cheese*   Sugar
Roasted peanuts

*These foods increase the production of mucus.

Home remedies

FEVER
* Chamomile tea. Limit two cups per day.

SORE THROAT
* Chew on sage leaf or drink sage tea.

CONGESTION
* Place a few drops of eucalyptus oil on child's sheet or covers or add to humidifier. This oil when inhaled eases congestion. Can also be used as a chest rub. But be sure to consult a knowledgeable professional as essential oils are strong and are absorbed into the skin quickly.

ACHES & PAINS
* A soothing bath - 2 cups of dried thyme added to 2 quarts of boiling water. Steep for 10 minutes. Drain and add to bath. Rest afterwards. This will sweat out the toxins.

CHILDREN'S ISSUES
Colic

Oftentimes it is milk-based formula that causes colic. Cow's milk is very hard to digest. Some doctors are now recommending no milk until 2 years of age.

 Herbs

These are the herbs that have been shown to help children suffering from colic.

Use these herbs to make tèas. Limit two cups per day.

Chamomile   Fennel
Catnip   Peppermint

Cloves are useful for reducing gas. Can use as a tea.

 Food

These are the foods that have been shown to aggravate colic.

Bananas   Cucumbers
Yogurt   Turnips
Lettuce   Green peppers
Garlic   Beans
Onions

Nursing mothers should also avoid these foods.

CHILDREN'S ISSUES

Colic

Home remedies

A HEATED SOLUTION
* ✳ Warm water in a hot water bottle can be placed on the child's abdomen.

A HANDS-ON APPROACH
* ✳ Massage before and after eating. Have child lie on back. Gently massage abdomen in a clockwise direction using two or three fingers.

Ear infections

That dreaded childhood affliction
that keeps us up all night.

Earaches are becoming one of the most common ailments for small children. Some practitioners believe that many children are allergic to cow's milk. This allergy can cause ear infections. Another problem is that parents are too quick to give children antibiotics which, if used improperly, can create strains of viruses that are resistant to treatment. This also diminishes the child's ability to form an immune system strong enough to fight viruses and bacteria. Lesson -- before going head-long into antibiotics, try testing for allergies or try alternative healing techniques.

CHILDREN'S ISSUES
Ear infections

 Home remedies

BLOW IT OFF
* For immediate relief, blow warm air, NOT HOT, from a hair dryer directly into the child's ear. Hold about six inches away. This can stop pain quickly.

GARLIC OIL
* Place a few drops in the child's ear. Here's how to make it. Crush 1 or 2 garlic cloves and place in ¼ cup of olive oil. Heat the mixture and then cool. Squeeze through a cheesecloth.

ECHINACEA
* For infections in general, Echinacea is an excellent herb. You might be able to find a chewable kind, or ask the health food store for a liquid tincture. I add it to the kids' juice. It really doesn't have a taste. (Or at least my kids know better than to complain!)

CHILDREN'S ISSUES

Diarrhea

Home remedies

THE WATER THAT BINDS
* The water than is left when you boil rice is an excellent home remedy for diarrhea. It is very binding.

THE BOUNTIFUL BEVERAGE - PEDIALYTE
* This drink replaces the electrolytes in the body that are lost due to the illness. If the child eats or drinks nothing else, this is the most important liquid to have.

DELIGHTFUL DRINKS
* Dissolve carob flour in pure water. Drink it every few hours.

* Drink a glass of barley water every few hours.

SOOTHING SNACKS
* Pretzels -- the salt is binding.

SIPPIN' TEAS
* Red raspberry, strawberry, peppermint, chamomile, slippery elm, oak bark.

CHILDREN'S ISSUES

Diarrhea

 A few more ideas

Again, my two cents. Learn the signs of dehydration. In young children age 5 and under, even a small amount of diarrhea can lead to dehydration.

Signs are: No tears when crying.
Dry lips.
No saliva.
Listlessness. (Too tired to get off of the couch even with the lure of candy!)
Non-responsive. (Doesn't seem able to answer basic questions.)

Try to catch the condition before dehydration. If you see the beginning of these signs go to your doctor. My wonderful doctor gave my daughter an IV and pumped her full of fluids to PREVENT her from becoming dehydrated and having to become hospitalized.

Circulation problems

∗ Combine ½ cup of rosemary and ½ cup of lavender to two quarts of water. Steep, strain and add to bath.

Cradle cap

∗ Vitamin E or almond oil rubbed into scalp.

Digestion problems

∗ Tea - chamomile, fennel, catnip, dill water.

CHILDREN'S ISSUES

Diaper rash

* Vitamin A and E - topically.

Dry skin

* Olive oil, almond oil, vitamin A, vitamin E, aloe vera gel.

Hyperactivity

* Keep children away from sweets, artificial flavoring, coloring, or preservatives.
* Vitamins that are helpful include:
  B-complex added to water or juice
  Vitamin D
  Calcium
  Multi-vitamin and mineral tablets

Stomach aches

* Herbal pillow filled with hops and chamomile is very relaxing for kids.
* Drink chamomile tea.
* A warm bath with yarrow will help reduce gas.

Teething

* Increase vitamin D and calcium.
* Drink catnip, peppermint, fennel, or chamomile tea.
* Rub gums with honey (add a little salt to honey).
* Rub peppermint oil on gums.
* SELKO method. Rub alcohol (whiskey or something strong) right onto the gum. It worked for all of the generations before me and it worked for my kids. Just don't tell your friends. Some people get so upset with me!

CHILDREN'S ISSUES

 ## A few more ideas

R ARELY FEED YOUR CHILDREN FAST FOOD! If I tell you all of the things that go into these foods, I'll make **myself** sick. Not to mention the undercooked meat and the lack of sanitary conditions at the restaurants.

If your kids want the latest toy, go to the toy store.

I believe that there is a connection between the mind and body. Therefore I tell my kids what I am giving them and why. They know that chicken soup or tea will get rid of their colds. I believe that they communicate this to their own internal intelligence system that governs the body.

Chapter
7
CIRCULATION PROBLEMS

Try to go
to more
parties.

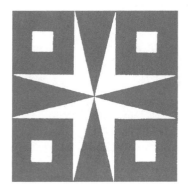

Every day for his 92 years, my great-grandfather drank a morning shot of whiskey. As young children we thought he just liked to drink. That was the only time we saw him take alcohol. Years later, he told us that he took it to help him with circulation problems. Well it worked. He was healthy and able to read the newspaper in 4 different languages until the day he died.

CIRCULATION PROBLEMS

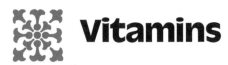 **Vitamins**

These are the vitamins that have been shown to help people suffering from circulation problems.

B Complex	C
B3	E
B6	Lecithin
B12	P
B15	

Food sources of Vitamins

Herb sources of Vitamins

B Complex
Apples, bananas, beets, cabbage, carrots, cauliflower, corn, grapefruit, kelp, liver, mushrooms, onions, oranges, peas, peanuts, potatoes, spinach, turnips, watercress, yeast.

B Complex
Kelp.

B3
Avocados, brewer's yeast, broccoli, carrots, cheese, corn flour, dates, eggs, figs, fish, kidney, liver, milk, meat (lean), peanuts (roasted), potatoes, poultry (white meat), prunes, tomatoes, wheat germ, whole wheat.

B3
Alfalfa, burdock, dandelion, fenugreek, kelp, parsley, sage.

B6
Avocados, bananas, brewer's

B6
Alfalfa.

CIRCULATION PROBLEMS

Food sources of Vitamins	*Herb sources of Vitamins*
yeast, cantaloupe, chicken, eggs, liver, kidney, milk, nuts, oats, peanuts, peas, potatoes, soybeans, vegetables (green leafy), walnuts, wheat bran, wheat germ.	

B12
Beef, cheese, clams, cottage cheese, eggs, fish, lamb, liver, kidney, milk, oysters, sardines, tofu.

B12
Alfalfa, kelp.

B15
Apricot kernels, brewer's yeast, brown rice (whole), pumpkin seeds, sesame seeds, whole grains.

C
Berries, black currants, broccoli, brussels sprouts, cabbage, cantaloupe, cauliflower, cherry juice (acerola), citrus fruits, guava, horseradish, kiwi, peppers (red, green), potatoes, rose hips, spinach, strawberries, tomatoes, turnips, watercress, vegetables (green leafy).

C
Alfalfa, burdock, boneset, catnip, capsicum, chickweed, dandelion, garlic, hawthorn, horseradish, kelp, parsley, plantain, papaya, rose hips, shepherd's purse, strawberry, watercress, yellow dock .

E
Broccoli, brown rice, brussels sprouts, cereals (whole grain),

E
Alfalfa, dandelion, gotu kola, kelp, raspberry, rose

CIRCULATION PROBLEMS

Food sources of Vitamins	**Herb sources of Vitamins**
corn, eggs, flour (enriched), liver, nuts, peas, soybeans, spinach, sweet potatotes, vegetables (green leafy), vegetable oil, wheat germ, whole wheat.	hips, watercress.

Lecithin
Corn, soybeans, vegetable oil, wheat germ oil.

P	**P**
Apricots, blackberries, black currants, buckwheat, cherries, citrus fruits (white skin and segment membranes), grapes, green peppers, plums, prunes, rose hips, spinach.	Dandelion, rose hips.

 # Herbs

These are the herbs that have been shown to help people suffering from circulation problems.

Echinacea	Dandelion	Hyssop
Red clover	Yellow dock	Pleurisy root
Burdock	Alfalfa	Rosemary
Myrrh	Licorice root	Lavender
Oregano	Ginkgo	Stinging nettle
Ginger	Cayenne	Rose hips

CIRCULATION PROBLEMS

Foods

These are the foods that have been shown to help people suffering with circulation problems.

Horseradish	Oat Bran	Onions
Garlic	Bananas	Pears
Fruit juices	Broccoli	Peas
Carrot juice	Brown rice	Spinach
Skins of citrus fruits	Lima beans	

These are the foods that have been shown to aggravate circulation problems.

Red meat	Coffee
White flour	Colas
White sugar	Spicy foods

Home remedies

THE VERSATILE HERB
* Hawthorn can both lower high blood pressure and raise low blood pressure.

STIMULATING BATHS
* Boil ½ cup of rosemary and ½ cup of lavender in 2 quarts of water. Simmer 15 minutes. Strain and add to bath. You can use this for a full bath, a foot bath, or an arm bath.

CIRCULATION PROBLEMS
Home remedies

HAND AND FOOT BATH
* Place sliced fresh ginger and 3 cinnamon sticks in 1 pint of water. Add Epsom salts and soak for 8 minutes both in the morning and in the evening.

CLEANSE YOUR BLOOD
* A fast consisting of fruit juice and carrot juice. (Consult a qualified person before attempting any type of fast.)

COLD FEET?
* Teas of cayenne, juniper or angelica can stimulate circulation.

MOVE IT
* Regular exercise.

THE NATURAL MASSAGE
* Using a natural bath brush or sponge, dry massage the entire body.

BRISK IDEA
* Dip a towel in cold water and rub it briskly over parts of the body.

Chapter

8

CONSTIPATION

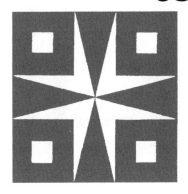

Ancient Egyptians never seemed to complain of this problem.

This modern day ailment is almost entirely due to poor diet and lack of exercise.

My cousin Barbara has figured out a way to continually re-educate herself in her field of family counseling, while maintaining regularity. Every morning she dons her walking shoes at 7:30 am. By the time she has reached the end of her driveway there are 3 people waiting for her. It seems they like to walk with Barbara as they can get her advice on their family problems and exercise all at the same time.

A brisk morning walk that conditions the abdominal muscles relieves constipation! Prevention is the key to this ailment. Eat a high fiber diet and exercise regularly.

CONSTIPATION

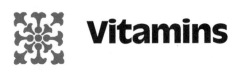 **Vitamins**

These are the vitamins that have been shown to help people suffering from constipation.

Acidophilus*	Folic acid	D
B complex	C	E
B 12		

*This is found in supplement form or in active yogurt cultures.

Food sources of Vitamins

Herb sources of Vitamins

B Complex
Apples, bananas, beans, beets, cabbage, carrots, cauliflower, corn, grapefruit, liver, mushrooms, onions, oranges, peas, peanuts, potatoes, spinach, turnips, watercress, yeast.

B Complex
Kelp.

B12
Beef, cheese, clams, cottage cheese, eggs, fish, lamb, liver, kidney, milk, oysters , sardines, tofu.

B12
Alfalfa, kelp.

B Factor: Folic Acid
Apricots, asparagus, avocados, beans, broccoli, carrots, cantaloupe, chick peas, egg yolks, flour (dark rye), liver, mushrooms, oranges, pumpkin, soy-

CONSTIPATION

Food sources of Vitamins

beans, spinach, sprouts, vegetables (green leafy), whole flour and wheat, yeast (tortula), yogurt.

C
Berries, black currants, broccoli, brussels sprouts, cabbage, cantaloupe, cauliflower, cherry juice (acerola), citrus fruits, guava, horseradish, kiwi, peppers (red green), potatoes, rose hips, spinach, strawberries, tomatoes, turnips, watercress, vegetables (green leafy).

D
Dairy, egg yolks, fish liver oils, herring, milk, salmon, spinach, tuna.

E
Broccoli, brown rice, brussels sprouts, cereal (whole grain), corn, eggs, flour (enriched), liver, nuts, peas, soybeans, spinach, sweet potatotes, vegetables (green leafy), vegetable oils, wheat germ, whole wheat.

Herb sources of Vitamins

C
Alfalfa, burdock, boneset, catnip, capsicum, chickweed, dandelion, garlic, hawthorn, horseradish, kelp, parsley, plantain, papaya, rose hips, shepherd's purse, strawberry, watercress, yellow dock.

D
Alfalfa, watercress.

E
Alfalfa, dandelion, gotu kola, kelp, raspberry, rose hips, watercress.

CONSTIPATION

 ## Herbs

These are the herbs that have been shown to help people suffering from constipation.

Cascara agrada	Dandelion	Barberry
Mallow	Fennel	Slippery elm
Aloe vera	Ginger	Mint
Basil	Burdock	Borage

 ## Food

These are the foods that have been shown to help people suffering from constipation.

Prunes	Dates	Sunflower
Brown rice	Apricots	Pumpkin seeds
Oats	Lemon	Pears
Barley	Apple	Apples
Wheat bran	Tomato	Fruit
Rice bran	Honey	Vegetables
Figs	Bee pollen	Green leafy vegetables

These are the foods have been shown to aggravate constipation.

Milk	Cheese	Caffeine

CONSTIPATION

Home remedies

DRINK AS THOUGH THE WORLD WERE ENDING
✳ 6-8 glasses per day of water, juice or tea.

NATURE'S HELPERS
✳ Two cascara sagrada capsules before bed. Use for 2-3 nights.

MASSAGE TECHNIQUE
✳ Two drops of essential oil of fennel massaged around the large intestine. Massage clockwise. If this strikes you as strange, our skin readily absorbs oil, sometimes faster than if we were to take the oil internally.

MORNING WAKE UP CALL
✳ First thing in the morning eat 5 pieces of dried fruit that you have left soaking in a cup of water overnight.
✳ Or stir 1 teaspoon to 1 tablespoon of cornmeal in a glass of cold water and drink immediately upon waking.

SQUARE DEAL
✳ Chop ½ pound each of figs, prunes and raisins. Mix with ½ cup of unprocessed bran. Place in shallow pan and cut into 1 tablespoon size squares. Wrap and store in refrigerator. Eat one square daily.

SEEDY IDEA
✳ Eat a handful of pumpkin and sunflower seeds.

WHATEVER HAPPENED TO CREAM CHEESE?
✳ Take several tablespoons of raw honey. Add bee pollen granules and spread on whole grain bread.

CONSTIPATION

 ## A few more ideas

Avoid laxatives, both natural and man made. Prolonged use of them is harmful. Laxatives should not be taken during pregnancy or nursing, or if you are taking chemical heart drugs.

Chapter
9

CUTS/BRUISES

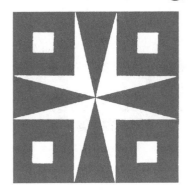

Quick! Take those hot cayenne peppers off the pizza and put them on your cuts and the bleeding will stop quickly. Plus, everyone will be so disgusted that you'll get to finish the pizza by yourself.

Recycle flowers. After you use them to brighten your yard and house make them into ointments to treat cuts and bruises.

The beautiful bright orange blossoms of the marigold plant contains an excellent ointment for cuts and bruises. Calendula (the family name for marigold) oil relieves inflammation and helps form new tissue.

Here's how to make it yourself. Place freshly harvested dry flower heads in a clear wide mouthed jar. Add cold vegetable oil to cover the flowers. Seal and let it sit 4-8 weeks. Shake once per day. When oil is a dark yellow color, press excess from flowers and filter through a sieve. Store in dark jar. This oil can be used for one year.

Cuts/Bruises

 # Vitamins

These are the vitamins that have been shown to help people suffering from cuts and bruises.

A	D
B Complex	E
B5	K
C	P

Food sources of Vitamins

A
Carrots, dairy, fish liver oil, fruits (yellow), lemon grass, liver, milk, margarine, okra, vegetables (green, yellow).

B Complex
Apples, bananas, beans, beets, cabbage, carrots, cauliflower, corn, grapefruit, liver, mushrooms, onions, oranges, peas, peanuts, potatoes, spinach, turnips, watercress, yeast.

B5
Beans, bran, brewer's yeast, chicken, eggs, fish (salt water), kidney, liver, molasses, nuts,

Herb sources of Vitamins

A
Alfalfa, burdock, capsicum, dandelion, garlic, kelp, marshmallow, papaya, parsley, raspberry, red clover, safflower, watercress, yellow dock.

B Complex
Kelp.

Cuts/Bruises

Food sources of Vitamins

Herb sources of Vitamins

pork, potatoes, tomatoes, vegetables (green), wheat germ, whole grains.

C

Berries, black currants, broccoli, brussels sprouts, cabbage, cantaloupe, cauliflower, cherry juice (acerola), citrus fruits, guava, horseradish, kiwi, peppers (red green), potatoes, rose hips, spinach, strawberries, tomatoes, turnips, watercress, vegetables (green leafy).

C

Alfalfa, burdock, boneset, catnip, capsicum, chickweed, dandelion, garlic, hawthorn, horseradish, kelp, parsley, plantain, papaya, rose hips, shepherd's purse, strawberry, watercress, yellow dock.

D

Dairy products, egg yolks, fish liver oil, herring, milk, salmon, spinach, tuna.

D

Alfalfa, watercress.

E

Broccoli, brown rice, brussels sprouts, cereals (whole grain), corn, eggs, flour (enriched), liver, nuts, peas, soybeans, spinach, sweet potatotes, vegetable oils, wheat germ, whole wheat.

E

Alfalfa, dandelion, gotu kola, kelp, raspberry, rose hips, watercress.

Cuts/Bruises

Food sources of Vitamins	*Herb sources of Vitamins*
K	**K**
Alfalfa, egg yolk, fish liver oils, legumes, liver, molasses (blackstrap), safflower oil, soybean oil, sprouts, vegetables (green leafy, root).	Alfalfa, kelp.
P	**P**
Apricots, blackberries, black currants, buckwheat, cherries, citrus fruits (white skin and segment membranes), grapes, green peppers, plums, prunes, rose hips, spinach.	Dandelion, rose hips.

 Herbs

These are the herbs that have been shown to help people suffering from cuts and bruises.

Calendula (topical)	Goldenseal	Cayenne
Echinacea	Dandelion	Sage
Plantain	Yarrow	

Cuts/Bruises

Food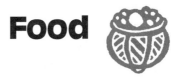

These are the foods that have been shown to help people suffering from cuts and bruises.

Citrus fruits   Green leafy vegetables   Pineapple juice

Home remedies

OIL RUB DOWN
* ✳ 2 teaspoons of essential oil of lavender or massage oil can be applied to cuts, bruises and bites.

JUICES FOR THE BRUISES
* ✳ For swelling due to bruises drink fresh pineapple juice. Or you can take the enzyme bromelain which is found in pineapples.

MAJOR LEAGUE MINOR CUTS
* ✳ To stop bleeding of minor cuts use any of the following:
  Goldenseal powder
  Cayenne pepper
  Moist tea leaves
  Aloe vera gel
  Papaya pulp

A SWELL IDEA
* ✳ To reduce swelling place a compress of hot pekoe tea. Or use 1 teaspoon of dried sage and ½ teaspoon of mint.

Cuts/Bruises

Home remedies

Place in boiling water. Steep 10 minutes. Add 1 table-spoon of apple cider vinegar. Saturate a towel in this combination and apply while still warm to the wound.

FLOWER POWER
* Calendula ointment (made from marigold flowers) heals small wounds and inhibits the inflammatory process. It can soothe pain and stimulate the supply of blood to skin.

KITCHEN REMEDY
* Moisten 2 tablespoon of dried oregano with hot water. Let stand covered for 10 minutes. Add more hot water to make a paste and apply to the area as a pain reliever.

NATURAL ANTISEPTICS
* Oil of clove, lavender and eucalyptus are antiseptics. If the cut is deep use St. John's Wort oil. To heal the cut apply vitamin E (in a gel form).

 A few more ideas

A homeopathic remedy that works is traumeel. Homeopathic remedies can be found at drugstores. The philosophy behind these treatments is that introducing an agent which causes the same symptoms as the illness allows the body to form antibodies to combat the illness.

Chapter
10

DIARRHEA

Run quickly
to the
refrigerator:
grab a yogurt.

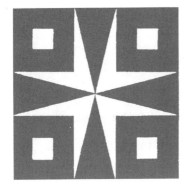

Did you think that the word acidophilus stamped on your cup of yogurt was really an aphrodisiac? And that's why nice looking people are always eating yogurt? Well, guess again.

Increasing our supply of acidophilus eases diarrhea.

Acidophilus is a bacteria found in the bowel and is present at birth. Its function is to protect us against such horrors as the now famous dangerous strains of E. coli bacteria. What is so interesting is that we are responsible for reducing our supply of acidophilus when we introduce any of the following into our bodies: antibiotics, coffee, birth control pills, excessive enemas, or large quantities of red meat.

DIARRHEA

 # Vitamins

These are the vitamins that have been shown to help people suffering from diarrhea.

Acidophilus*	B3
B Complex	Folic acid
B 1	C

*This is found in supplement form or in active yogurt cultures.

Food sources of Vitamins

B Complex
Apples, bananas, beans, beets, cabbage, carrots, cauliflower, corn, grapefruit, liver, mushrooms, onions, oranges, peas, peanuts, potatoes, spinach, turnips, watercress, yeast.

B1
Beans (dried), blackstrap molasses, bran, brewer's yeast, cereal grains (unrefined), egg yolks, milk, oatmeal, peanuts, peas, pork (lean), prunes, raisins, rice husks, vegetables, wheat germ, whole wheat.

Herb sources of Vitamins

B Complex
Kelp.

B1
Capsicum, dandelion, fenugreek, kelp, safflower, watercress.

DIARRHEA

Food sources of Vitamins

B3

Avocados, brewer's yeast, broccoli, carrots, cheese, corn flour, dates, eggs, figs, fish, kidney, liver, milk, meat (lean), peanuts (roasted), potatoes, poultry (white meat), prunes, tomatoes, wheat germ, whole wheat.

B Factor: Folic Acid

Apricots, asparagus, avocados, beans, broccoli, carrots, cantaloupe, chick peas, egg yolks, flour (dark rye), liver, mushrooms, oranges, pumpkin, soybeans, spinach, sprouts, vegetables (green leafy), whole flour and wheat, yeast (tourtula), yogurt.

C

Berries, black currants, broccoli, brussels sprouts, cabbage, cantaloupe, cauliflower, cherry juice (acerola), citrus fruits, guava, horseradish, kiwi, peppers (red, green), potatoes, rose hips, spinach, strawberries, tomatoes, turnips, watercress, vegetables (green leafy).

Herb sources of Vitamins

B3

Alfalfa, burdock, dandelion, fenugreek, kelp, parsley, sage.

C

Alfalfa, burdock, boneset, catnip, capsicum, chickweed, dandelion, garlic, hawthorn, horseradish, kelp, parsley, plantain, papaya, rose hips, shepherd's purse, strawberry, watercress, yellow dock.

DIARRHEA

 ## Herbs

These are the herbs that have been shown to help people suffering from diarrhea.

Basil	Cayenne	Kelp	Sage
Blackberry	Fenugreek	Marigold	Slippery elm
Bayberry	Garlic	Peppermint	Thyme
Chamomile	Ginger	Raspberry	Yarrow
Cinnamon			

 ## Food

These are the foods that have been shown to help people suffering from diarrhea.

Blueberries	Oat bran	Legumes	Root vegetables:
Dried apples	Rice bran	Honey	carrots,
Starchy soup	Black currants	Barley	potatoes,
Cereal	Bananas	Nutmeg	turnips, etc.
Yogurt	Beans		

These are the foods have been shown to aggravate diarrhea.

Milk	Sweets	Whole grain cereal
Juice	Fruit	High fibre, bulky foods
Diluted soup		

DIARRHEA

Home remedies

RICE WATER -THE LATEST TREND
* Cook brown rice and save the water. It is very binding.

FOR ADULTS ONLY
* Half teaspoon of fenugreek seeds with water. Three times daily. It's a quick relief.

SMASHING SUCCESS
* Eat mashed raw bananas.

CARROT SOUP
* Cook 1 pound of carrots. Put in blender with 1 cup of water and ¾ teaspoon of salt. Add enough water to make a quart of soup and heat. Take small amounts every half hour until better.

BLACKBERRY JUICE
* Add ½ teaspoon of cayenne and ¼ teaspoon of nutmeg to 1 cup of blackberry juice. Drink ¼ cup every few hours.

EGGZACTLY CORRECT
* Combine 1 egg white with the juice of one lemon. Beat until frothy. Pour over chipped ice and eat with a spoon. (Be sure to keep your pinky up.)

BACK TO BASICS
* Sip strong hot lemonade every 30 minutes.

FOR PREVENTION
* Add dill (an herb) to your diet.

DIARRHEA

 A few more ideas

Diarrhea is caused when the mucous membrane within the bowel becomes irritated or inflamed and fails to absorb liquid from food material.

Some reasons for irritation (aside from family arguments) are allergies, antibiotic medications, bacterial infections, fatigue, food poisoning, nutritional deficiencies and, as always, stress.

When traveling, less than hygienic conditions coupled with unfamiliar bacterial flora can cause diarrhea. Before meals, try taking lemon or lime juice. Taking three acidophilus capsules during each meal has been known to help.

Massage to the rescue. Using deep thumb pressure, massage the abdomen. The spot is located 1 1/2 inches directly below the navel. Another location is just below the kneecap to the outside of the shinbone.

Chapter
11
DIZZINESS/ NAUSEA

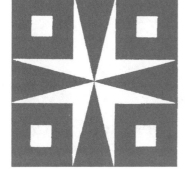

To cure dizziness one must eat organ meats, the mere sound of which makes most people nauseous.

Here are some other digestible solutions.

S tacy, another cousin (good thing for me I have such a sick family), was always apprehensive about traveling. It was not the fear of flying or driving or even falling off a ship, it was the dizzy feeling she always got when traveling. Thanks to the healing powers of ginger pills, Stacy is now an airline stewardess. Not really, but the change is miraculous. Half an hour prior to traveling she takes 2 pills and then a couple more every 4 hours. She also uses ginger at any other time she feels dizzy, whether due to illness or just her natural tendency toward dizziness.

DIZZINESS

 Vitamins

These are the vitamins that have been shown to help people suffering from dizziness.

B Complex	Choline
B3	C
B6	E
B15	P

Food sources of Vitamins

B Complex
Apples, bananas, beans, beets, cabbage, carrots, cauliflower, corn, grapefruit, liver, mushrooms, onions, oranges, peas, peanuts, potatoes, spinach, turnips, watercress, yeast.

B3
Avocados, brewer's yeast, broccoli, carrots, cheese, corn flour, dates, eggs, figs, fish, kidney, liver, milk, meat (lean), peanuts (roasted), potatoes, poultry (white meat), prunes, tomatoes, wheat germ, whole wheat.

Herb sources of Vitamins

B Complex
Kelp.

B3
Alfalfa, burdock, dandelion, fenugreek, kelp, parsley, sage.

DIZZINESS

Food sources of Vitamins

B6
Avocados, banana, brewer's yeast, cantaloupe, chicken, eggs, liver, kidney, milk, nuts, oats, peanuts, peas, potatoes, soybeans, vegetables (green leafy), walnuts, wheat bran, wheat germ.

B15
Apricot kernels, brewer's yeast, brown rice (whole), pumpkin seeds, sesame seeds, whole grains.

B Factor: Choline
Brain, brewer's yeast, egg yolks, fish, heart, liver, peas, peanut butter, seeds, soybeans, turnip, vegetables (green leafy), wheat germ.

C
Berries, black currants, broccoli, brussels sprouts, cabbage, cantaloupe, cauliflower, cherry juice (acerola), citrus fruits, guava, horseradish, kiwi, peppers (red, green).

Herb sources of Vitamins

B6
Alfalfa, burdock, boneset, catnip, capsicum, chickweed, dandelion, garlic, hawthorn, horseradish, kelp, parsley, plantain, papaya, rose hips, shepherd's purse, strawberry, watercress, yellow dock.

DIZZINESS

Food sources of Vitamins	Herb sources of Vitamins
E	**E**
Broccoli, brown rice, brussels sprouts, cereals (whole grain), corn, eggs, flour (enriched), liver, nuts, peas, soybeans, spinach, sweet potatoes, vegetables (green leafy), vegetable oils, wheat germ, whole wheat.	Alfalfa, dandelion, gotu kola, kelp, raspberry, rose hips, watercress.
P	**P**
Apricots, blackberries, black currants, buckwheat, cherries, citrus fruits (white skin and segment membranes), grapes, peppers (green), plums, prunes, rose hips, spinach.	Dandelion, rose hips, potatoes, rose hips, spinach, strawberries, tomatoes, turnips, watercress, vegetables (green leafy).

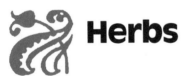 **Herbs**

These are the herbs that have been shown to help people suffering from dizziness.

Ginger   Rosemary
Ginkgo   Echinacea

DIZZINESS

Food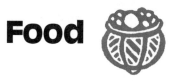

These are the foods that have been shown to help people suffering from dizziness.

Orange juice	Dried fruits	Pasta
Foods containing iron	Liver	Peas
Dried beans	Lean red meat	Potatoes
Cereals	Nuts	Green leafy
Whole grain & enriched bread		vegetables

These are the foods that have been shown to aggravate dizziness.

Hot spicy foods	Citrus fruits
Sour-tasting food	Caffeine
Salt	

Home remedies

GINGER PILLS TO THE RESCUE
* Take 2 capsules when you feel dizzy. They're effective for 4 hours. Take ½ hour prior to traveling, if travel makes you dizzy.

A POWERFUL POTION
* Put a freshly cut onion in a plastic bag and inhale the fumes. If you don't pass out it can help dizziness.

A QUICK DRINK
* 1 glass of orange juice should stop that funny feeling.

NAUSEA

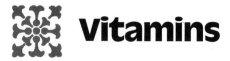 **Vitamins**

These are the vitamins that have been shown to help people suffering from nausea.

B6
C

Food sources of Vitamins	*Herb sources of Vitamins*
B6	**B6**
Avocados, bananas, brewer's yeast, cantaloupe, chicken, eggs, liver, kidney, molasses, nuts, pork, potatoes, tomatoes, vegetables (green), wheat germ, whole grains.	Alfalfa.
C	**C**
Berries, black currants, broccoli, brussels sprouts, cabbage, cantaloupe, cauliflower, cherry juice (acerola), citrus fruits, guava, horseradish, kiwi, peppers (red, green), potatoes, rose hips, spinach, strawberries, tomatoes, turnips, watercress, vegetables (green leafy).	Alfalfa, burdock, boneset, catnip, capsicum, chickweed, dandelion, garlic, hawthorn, horseradish, kelp, parsley, plantain, papaya, rose hips, shepherd's purse, strawberry leaf, watercress, yellow dock.

NAUSEA

Herbs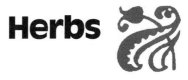

These are the herbs that have been shown to help people suffering from nausea.

Ginger	Yarrow	Peppermint
Goldenseal	Chamomile	Cayenne
Mint	Fennel	Hops

Food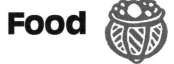

These are the foods that have been shown to help people suffering from nausea.

Soup with ground red pepper	Cucumber	Oranges
Apples - raw, shredded	Raspberries	Celery
with honey	Ginger ale	Barley
(Apples & Honey, now that		
sounds familiar)		

NAUSEA

 # Home remedies

A SPOT OF TEA
* Yarrow tea can stop the nausea quickly. Clove tea works, or add 2 teaspoons of ground cloves to 1 cup of milk.

YET ANOTHER USE FOR BAKING SODA
* One tablespoon of baking soda to 1 glass of water.

WRIST BAND
* Found at maternity stores or sometimes called sailor's bands, these bands put pressure on that point of the wrist that controls nausea. It works on the same principle as acupuncture.

CONTINUOUS DRINKING
* Add 1 tablespoon of apple cider vinegar to water. Drink 1 tablespoon every 5 minutes until you feel better. Then drink 1 tablespoon every 15 minutes.

CHEW ON THIS
* Chew fresh sprigs of mint,
    or ½ teaspoon of dry grated grapefruit peel,
    or small pieces of bread,
    or clove.

IT'S GINGER AGAIN
* Place 4 quarter-sized slices of ginger in boiling water. Steep for 10 minutes and strain. Drink hot.

NAUSEA

Home Remedies

LAY IT ON ME

∗ On your bare stomach place fresh peppermint leaves that have been crushed. Secure them in place and stay seated. Don't lie down.

DIZZINESS/NAUSEA

 # A few more ideas

B ee propolis, which is the substance that is collected by bees from cone-bearing trees, is used to treat dizziness. This substance also oozes from the trees. Bee propolis stimulates the immune system.

A Chinese remedy for dizziness is fresh celery juice mixed with honey. Celery has a mild sedative effect.

Chapter
12

EARACHES

Too much talk,
not enough
action.

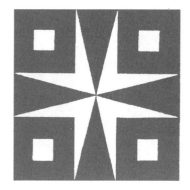

My friend Cindy has actually used this method to cure an earache. She peels a clove of garlic, cuts the hard ends and tapes the remainder to the inside of her ear-lobe. She says you do get used to the odor.

Earaches are becoming one of the most common ailments for small children. Some practitioners believe that many children are allergic to cow's milk. This allergy can cause ear infections. Another problem is that parents are too quick to give children antibiotics which, if used improperly, can create strains of viruses that are resistant to treatment. This also diminshes the child's ability to form an immune system strong enough to fight viruses and bacteria. Before going headlong into antibiotics, try testing for allergies or try alternative healing techniques.

EARACHES

 Vitamins

These are the vitamins that have been shown to help people suffering from earaches.

A	B Complex	C
Acidophilus*	B6	E
Beta-carotene		

*This is found in supplement form or in active yogurt cultures.

Food sources of Vitamins

A
Carrots, dairy, fish liver oil, fruits (yellow), lemon grass, liver, milk, margarine, okra, vegetables (green, yellow).

Beta-carotene
Apricots, broccoli, cantaloupe, collard greens, kale, mangoes, papayas, peppers, pumpkin, peaches, romaine lettuce, spinach, squash, sweet potatoes, tropical fruit.

Herb sources of Vitamins

A
Alfalfa, burdock, capsicum, dandelion, garlic, kelp, marshmallow, papaya, parsley, raspberry, red clover, safflower, watercress, yellow dock.

Betacarotene
Bay leaves (crumbled), basil, marjoram, parsley, sage.

EARACHES

Food sources of Vitamins

Herb sources of Vitamins

B Complex
Apples, bananas, beans, beets, cabbage, carrots, cauliflower, corn, grapefruit, liver, mushrooms, onions, oranges, peas, peanuts, potatoes, spinach, turnips, watercress, yeast.

B Complex
Kelp.

B6
Avocados, bananas, brewer's yeast, cantaloupe, chicken, eggs, liver, kidney, milk, nuts, oats, peanuts, peas, potatoes, soybeans, vegetables (green leafy), walnuts, wheat bran, wheat germ.

B6
Alfalfa.

C
Berries, black currants, broccoli, brussels sprouts, cabbage, cantaloupe, cauliflower, cherry juice (acerola), citrus fruits, guava, horseradish, kiwi, peppers (red, green), potatoes, rose hips, spinach, strawberries, tomatoes, turnips, watercress, vegetables (green leafy).

C
Alfalfa, burdock, boneset, catnip, capsicum, chickweed, dandelion, garlic, hawthorn, horseradish, kelp, parsley, plantain, papaya, rose hips, shepherd's purse, strawberry, watercress, yellow dock.

EARACHES

Food sources of Vitamins	*Herb sources of Vitamins*
E Broccoli, brown rice, brussels sprouts, cereals (whole grain), corn, eggs, flour (enriched), liver, nuts, peas, soybeans, spinach, sweet potatoes, vegetables (green leafy), vegetable oils, wheat germ, whole wheat.	**E** Alfalfa, dandelion, gotu kola, kelp, raspberry, rose hips, watercress.

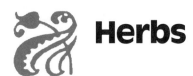 **Herbs**

These are the herbs that have been shown to help people suffering from earaches.

Ginkgo - good for
    ringing in ears
St. Johns wort oil
Mullein oil

Garlic oil
Echinacea
Chamomile
Slippery elm

EARACHES

Food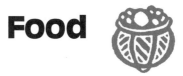

These are the foods that have been shown to help people suffering from earaches.

Yogurt - with an active culture (acidophilus)	Fresh fruit Vegetables juices	Potatoes

These are the foods that have been shown to aggravate earaches:

Dairy products
Junk food
Meat

For children.
Avoid milk, wheat products, and eggs. Studies show that allergies to these products can cause chronic ear infections that may lead to eventual hearing loss.

EARACHES

 # Home remedies

POUR IT ON
* Here are a few types of oil that are poured into the ear using a dropper. Only a few drops are necessary.

  Garlic oil
  Heat 2 cloves of garlic in olive oil. Remove garlic and use remaining oil.

  St. John's wort oil
  You can purchase this as a ready made oil. It has been used for many, many years.

  Bee pollen
  Warm the granules.

PRESS IT ON
* Soak a cloth in chamomile or slippery elm tea. Apply to the ear and cover it with a dry cloth.

TIE IT ON
* Take a sliced roasted onion and tie it over the ear.

* Heat table salt. Wrap in a cloth and tie it under the ear while resting the head on a pillow.

EARACHES

Home Remedies

SOAK IT
* Make a mustard foot bath. Use 3-4 cups of warm water and add 1 tablespoon of mustard powder. This draws the blood away from the head. If the earache is severe you can make a mustard plaster using 3 tablespoons of flour to 1 tablespoon of mustard powder. Add water to make a paste and place on gauze. Put a little oil on the skin behind the ear and cover with the gauze with the paste on it.

AND GARGLE
* Using saltwater, gargle at the first sign of an earache. This brings more blood to the eustachian tube and helps fight infection.

EARACHES

 A few more ideas

A particularly pleasant eardrop formula is made from fresh peppermint juice. Here's how to do it. Take fresh leaves and pound on them to squeeze out the juice. A few drops of this potion, directly into the ear is all it should take to ease an earache.

Chapter

13

ECZEMA

This ailment
gets
under
your skin.

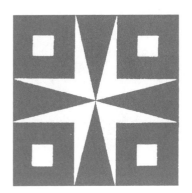

Megan's daughter was never seen without gloves. In this day and age this formality might seem out of place. However in her case, gloves provided the necessary protection from eczema. Her young daughter could hardly be expected to refrain from scratching the exasperating results of eczema. But scratching led to infection. Luckily as she grew older, the eczema passed and she now only wears gloves for fashion's sake.

ECZEMA

 Vitamins

These are the vitamins that have been shown to help people suffering from eczema.

A	Inositol	F
B Complex	C	P
B3	E	PABA

Food sources of Vitamins

Herb sources of Vitamins

A

Carrots, dairy, fish liver oil, fruits (yellow), lemon grass, liver, milk, margarine, okra, vegetables (green, yellow).

A

Alfalfa, burdock, capsicum, dandelion, garlic, kelp, marshmallow, papaya, parsley, raspberry, red clover, safflower, watercress, yellow dock.

B Complex

Apples, bananas, beans, beets, cabbage, carrots, cauliflower, corn, grapefruit, liver, mushrooms, onions, oranges, peas, peanuts, potatoes, spinach, turnips, watercress, yeast.

B Complex

Kelp.

B3

Avocados, brewer's yeast, broccoli, carrots, cheese, corn

B3

Alfalfa, burdock, dandelion, fenugreek, kelp, parsley, sage.

ECZEMA

Food sources of Vitamins	*Herb sources of Vitamins*

flour, dates, eggs, figs, fish, kidney, liver, milk, meat (lean), peanuts (roasted), potatoes, poultry (white meat), prune, tomatoes, wheat germ, whole wheat.

B Factor: Inositol
Beans (dried lima), brains, brewer's yeast, cabbage, cantaloupe, grapefruit, heart, liver, molasses, oatmeal, oranges, peanuts, raisins, sesame seeds, soybeans, wheat germ, whole wheat bread.

C
Berries, black currants, broccoli, brussels sprouts, cabbage, cantaloupe, cauliflower, cherry juice (acerola), citrus fruits, guava, horseradish, kiwi, peppers (red, green), potatoes, rose hips, spinach, strawberries, tomatoes, turnips, vegetables (green, leafy).

C
Alfalfa, burdock, boneset, catnip, capsicum, chickweed, dandelion, garlic, hawthorn, horseradish, kelp, parsley, plantain, papaya, rose hips, shepherd's purse, strawberry, watercress, yellow dock.

E
Broccoli, brown rice, brussels sprouts, cereals (whole grain), corn, eggs, flour (enriched), kidney, liver, nuts, rich (brown), peas, soybeans, spin-

E
Alfalfa, dandelion, gotu kola, kelp, raspberry, rose hips, watercress.

ECZEMA

Food sources of Vitamins

Herb sources of Vitamins

ach, sweet potatoes, vegetables (green leafy), vegetable oils, wheat germ, whole wheat.

F

Almonds, avocados, black currant oil, cod liver oil, corn oil, cottonseed oil, flaxseed oil, linseed oil, peanuts, pecans, primrose oil, safflower oil, sunflower oil, soybean, wheat germ.

P

Apricots, blackberries, black currants, buckwheat, cherries, citrus fruits (white skin and segment membranes), grapes, peppers (green), plums, prunes, rose hips, spinach.

P

Dandelion, rose hips.

PABA

Bran, brewer's yeast, molasses, organ meats (kidney), rice, wheat germ, whole grains.

ECZEMA

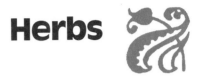

Herbs

These are the herbs that have been shown to help people suffering from eczema.

Chamomile
Catnip
Marjoram
Slippery elm

Burdock
Blueberry
Hawthorn

Strawberry leaf
Echinacea
St. John's wort oil

Food

These are the foods that have been shown to help people suffering from eczema.

Yogurt with acidophilus - 1 per day
Raw potato - 1 per day
Watercress
Green leafy vegetables

Sprouts
Celery
Pineapple
Grapes
Melons

Kelp
Unsalted seeds
Onions
Papayas
Pears

Juices { Spinach
Lettuce
Celery
Alfalfa

ECZEMA

Food

These are the foods that have been shown to aggravate eczema:

Shellfish Chocolate Wheat products such as rice
Citrus fruits Sweets Rye
Orange juice Flavorings Millet and barley (if allergic
Dairy products Preservatives to wheat products)

The following foods can cause reactions:

Eggs Honey Berries
Chicken Bananas Tomatoes

 Home remedies

SMOOTH OVER THAT ITCHY FEELING
 * Calendula cream for dry skin and to soothe soreness.
   Aloe vera cream. St. John's Wort oil.
   (NOTE: Don't apply cortisone cream unless eczema
   is very serious. It helps the symptoms but pushes the
   poisons back into the body.)

JUMP OUT OF YOUR SKIN
 * Chamomile bath- Prepare one cup of tea and place into
   bath to relieve itching.
WEEP NO MORE
 * For weeping eczema- avoid applying powders and
   pastes. Apply a moist compress until the acute phase
   has passed.

ECZEMA

Home remedies

COMPRESS YOURSELF
* Chamomile compress- Using a linen or flannel cloth, or gauze bandage, saturate with warm chamomile tea and apply to area until cool.
* Brewer's yeast compress - Mix 1 to 6 tablespoons of brewer's yeast with water and pat over affected area.

JUST A TUB OF FUN
* Colloidal oatmeal baths
* Baking Soda Tub- 1-1 1/2 cups of baking soda in a warm tub.
* Cornstarch Tub - First place 2 cups of cornstarch in tub. Add water.
* Oily Tub - Add 1 tablespoon of vegetable oil to bath.
* Last Tub -1 cup of vinegar.

DON'T LET IT RUB YOU THE WRONG WAY
* Garlic - Mash raw garlic and rub on area.
* Potato - Grate raw potato and rub on area.
* Vinegar - Sponge area with 1 tablespoon of apple cider vinegar in 1 cup water. Rub on area.

TAKE A LOOK INSIDE
* Primrose oil is a good source of the fatty acid that might be lacking.

ECZEMA

 A few more ideas

Use a deodorant instead of an antiperspirant. Antiperspirants contain aluminum chloride which can irritate sensitive skin.

Metal jewelry with nickel in it can cause eczema.

Don't use colored tissue paper or toilet paper.

Chapter
14

EYE PROBLEMS

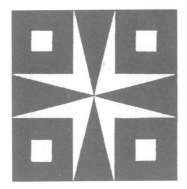

Relief in sight
for sore eyes.

Beta-carotene - the active ingredient in a carrot really does work. It is the primary chemical that your system converts into Vitamin A.

Other Sources of beta-carotene are: apricots, broccoli, cantaloupe, collar greens, kale, mangos, papayas, peppers, pumpkin, peaches, romaine lettuce, spinach, squash, sweet potatoes, tropical fruits.

Herbal sources are : bay leaves (crumbled), basil, marjoram, parsley, and sage.

Spices include: cumin, curry, paprika, oregano, and tarragon.

EYE PROBLEMS

 Vitamins

These are the vitamins that have been shown to help people suffering from eye problems.

A	B12	D
B Complex	Inositol	E
B2	C	

Food sources of Vitamins

A
Carrots, dairy, fish liver oil, fruits (yellow), lemon grass, liver, milk, margarine, okra, vegetables (green, yellow).

B Complex
Apples, bananas, beans, beets, cabbage, carrots, cauliflower, corn, grapefruit, liver, mushrooms, onions, oranges, peas, peanuts, potatoes, spinach, turnips, watercress, yeast.

B2
Avocados, beans, brewer's yeast, cheese, currants, eggs, fish, kidney, liver, milk, molasses, nuts, vegetables (green leafy).

Herb sources of Vitamins

A
Alfalfa, burdock, capsicum, dandelion, garlic, kelp, marshmallow, papaya, parsley, raspberry, red clover, safflower, watercress, yellow dock.

B Complex
Kelp.

EYE PROBLEMS

Food sources of Vitamins

B12
Beef, cheese, clams, cottage cheese, eggs, fish, lamb, liver, kidney, milk, oysters, sardines, tofu.

B Factor: Inositol
Beans (dried lima), brains, brewer's yeast, cabbage, cantaloupe, grapefruit, heart, liver, molasses, oatmeal, oranges, peanuts, raisins, sesame seeds, soybeans, wheat germ, whole wheat bread.

C
Berries, black currants, broccoli, brussels sprouts, cabbage, cantaloupe, cauliflower, cherry juice (acerola), citrus fruits, guava, horseradish, kiwi, peppers (red, green), potatoes, rose hips, spinach, strawberries, tomatoes, turnips, watercress, vegetables (green leafy).

D
Dairy, egg yolks, fish liver oils, herring, milk, salmon, spinach, tuna.

Herb sources of Vitamins

B12
Alfalfa, kelp.

C
Alfalfa, burdock, boneset, catnip, capsicum, chickweed, dandelion, garlic, hawthorn, horseradish, kelp, parsley, plantain, papaya, rose hips, shepherd's purse, strawberry, watercress, yellow dock.

D
Alfalfa, watercress.

EYE PROBLEMS

Food sources of Vitamins

E
Broccoli, brown rice, brussels sprouts, cereals (whole grain), corn, eggs, flour (enriched), kidney, liver, nuts, peas, soybeans, spinach, sweet potatoes, vegetables (green leafy), vegetable oils, wheat germ, whole wheat.

Herb sources of Vitamins

E
Alfalfa, dandelion, gotu kola, kelp, raspberry, rose hips, watercress.

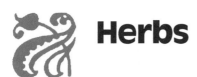 **Herbs**

These are the herbs that have been shown to help people suffering from eye problems.

Fennel
Goldenseal
Bayberry

Red raspberry
Cayenne
Lemon grass

EYE PROBLEMS

Food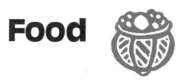

These are the foods that have been shown to help people suffering from eye problems.

Carrots	Liver	Fresh fruit
Broccoli	Cod liver oil	Sunflower seeds
Cauliflower	Squash	Yogurt
Raw cabbage	Green vegetables	Watercress

These are the foods that have been shown to aggravate eye problems:

Spicy foods	Alcohol
Sugar	Coffee

Home remedies

BLOODSHOT EYES

VITAMINS TO THE RESCUE
* Vitamins A, E, and B complex can correct bloodshot eyes.

POTATO PRESS
* Grate an unpeeled white potato. (Wash, of course.) Place a large spoonful directly on the eyelid. Cover with a gauze pad and let sit for 1-2 hours. Can also use cooked mashed beets.

EYE PROBLEMS

Home remedies

EYESTRAIN

BAT YOUR EYES
* Frequent blinking helps.

IMAGERY
* Sitting at a table, place the palms of your hands over your eyes. Place lightly and do not put any pressure on the eyeballs. Imagine a black box lined with velvet. This imagery helps restore normal vision.

SUN SALUTE
* Sit in the sun with your eyes closed. To ensure that your entire eyelids are bathed in sunlight, turn your head from side to side. Try this method a few minutes over a 3 week period. Next try a quick blink while sitting in the sun.

CUCUMBER PRESS
* Place sliced cucumbers on your eyes.

EYE PROBLEMS

Home remedies

IRRITATED EYES

COMFORTING COMPRESS
* Saturate a few cloths with hot water. Alternate cloths every 5 minutes. Make compresses from either chamomile, fennel or rosemary tea.

RELAX, LIE DOWN
* With your feet raised higher than your head, lie down for 15 minutes.

THE RETURN OF THE POTATO
* This time use a raw red potato. Keep on eyelid for 20 minutes.

EYE PROBLEMS

 A few more ideas

Cooled tea bags, especially herbal tea bags, offer relief for red and itchy eyes. It is the tannic acid contained in the tea bags that is the active agent of healing.

For general eye problems, boil cabbage leaves until limp. Remove leaves, drain water, and make a poultice from the leaves.

A sweeter poultice would be 1 teaspoon of honey mixed with water. Simmer for 5 minutes. Dip a cloth in the solution and apply to the eye.

Chapter
15

GUM PROBLEMS

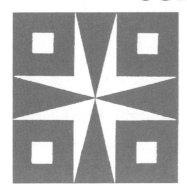

Open up the
aluminum foil .....
Seriously,
gum problems
can become
severe,
so it's best
to conquer them
at the first sign of
trouble.

I begged, I pleaded, I bribed, but no one would discuss their gum problems with me. So I'll testify to hearsay. The herb myrrh has been used since the Tang Dynasty (600 AD) to heal wounds, especially in the mouth.

Baking soda too is a healing agent, so after you have deodorized your refrigerator, cleaned your tub, and applied to mosquito bites, just go ahead and use the baking soda on your gums and teeth.

GUM PROBLEMS

 Vitamins

These are the vitamins that have been shown to help people suffering from gum problems.

A	C	P
B Complex	E	
B3		

Food sources of Vitamins

Herb sources of Vitamins

A
Carrots, dairy, fish liver oil, fruits (yellow), lemon grass, liver, milk, .margarine, okra, vegetables (green, yellow).

A
Alfalfa, burdock, capsicum, dandelion, garlic, kelp, marshmallow, papaya, parsley, raspberry, red clover, safflower, watercress, yellow dock.

B Complex
Apples, bananas, beans, beets, cabbage, carrots, cauliflower, corn, grapefruit, liver, mushroom, onions, oranges, peas, peanuts, potatoes, spinach, turnips, watercress, yeast.

B Complex
Kelp.

B3
Avocado, brewer's yeast, broccoli, carrots, cheese, corn flour, dates, eggs, figs, fish, kidney, liver, milk, molasses, nuts, vegetables (green leafy).

B3
Alfalfa, burdock, dandelion, fenugreek, kelp, parsley, sage.

GUM PROBLEMS

Food sources of Vitamins	*Herb sources of Vitamins*
C	**C**
Berries, black currants, broccoli, brussels sprouts, cabbage, cantaloupe, cauliflower, cherry juice (acerola), citrus fruits, guava, horseradish, kiwi, peppers (red, green), potatoes, rose hips, spinach, strawberries, tomatoes, turnips, vegetables (green leafy), watercress.	Alfalfa, burdock, boneset, catnip, capsicum, chickweed, dandelion, garlic, hawthorn, horseradish, kelp, parsley, plantain, papaya, rose hips, shepherd's purse, strawberry, watercress, yellow dock.
E	**E**
Broccoli, brown rice, brussels sprouts, cereals (whole grain), corn, eggs, flour(enriched), kidney, liver, nuts, peas, soybeans, spinach, sweet potatoes, vegetables (green leafy), vegetable oils, wheat germ, whole wheat.	Alfalfa, dandelion, gotu kola, kelp, raspberry, rose hips, watercress.
P	**P**
Apricots, blackberries, black currants, buckwheat, cherries, citrus fruits (white skin and segment membranes), grapes, peppers (green), plums, prunes, rose hips, spinach.	Dandelion, rose hips.

GUM PROBLEMS

 ## Herbs

These are the herbs that have been shown to help people suffering from gum problems.

Echinacea
Goldenseal
Bayberry

Myrrh - Do not
use during pregnancy

 ## Food

These are the foods that have been shown to help people suffering from gum problems.

Fresh fruit
Green leafy vegetables
Meat

Whole grains
Brussels sprouts

Raw cauliflower
Watercress

These are the foods have been shown to aggravate gum problems:

Sweets

GUM PROBLEMS

Home remedies

HOW MOTHER NATURE FIGHTS PLAQUE
* Mix 1 tablespoon of apple cider vinegar in a glass of water. Rinse mouth. This removes plaque and tartar, the cause of many gum problems.
* Use these three teas as mouthwash Chamomile, Sage, Red raspberry.

GOT ME WORKING DAY AND NIGHT
* In the morning apply witch hazel extract.
  In the evening apply oil of eucalyptus.

TOOTHPASTE WITH A BITE
* Brush with goldenseal herb power daily for a month. Change your toothpaste and your toothbrush monthly. Try different brands to prevent irritation.

RUBDOWN
* Rub vitamin E oil on inflamed gums.

RUB SALT IN THE WOUND
* Massage gums with a rough cloth. Then massage with salt.

WHERE FIGS DARE NOT ROAM
* Cook figs in milk. Then rub on sore gums. Next drink the liquid. (Be sure to see the section on indigestion.)

GUM PROBLEMS

Home remedies

IT JUST FEELS GOOD

* Hydrogen peroxide fights plaque and all those other lovely things that gather on your gums. Dilute the hydrogen peroxide to 35% and make a solution of ½ water and ½ hydrogen peroxide. Swish and brush. Try a few drops at first to get used to this solution.

 A few more ideas

Gingivitis, pyorrhea ... the mere mention of these diseases sends shudders down our spines. These are periodontal diseases that cause our gums to bleed (gingivitis) or manifest as infections between the gum and tooth area (pyorrhea). Not to worry, increase your intake of Vitamin C and calcium. Use proper dental hygiene and you can kiss those diseases good-bye.

Chapter
16

HEADACHES

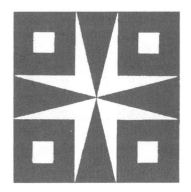

The throbbing,
the pounding,
the searing pain.
And that's just a
family political
discussion.

M y cousin Dubby has found an easy cure for her migraines. She no longer listens to the news. Seriously, she chews on fresh feverfew leaves at the start of a migraine. Feverfew is the long standing cure for migraines. Some people chew the leaves on a daily basis. Others find the leaves can cause irritation and use feverfew tea instead.

HEADACHES

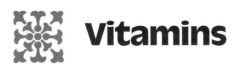 **Vitamins**

These are the vitamins that have been shown to help people suffering from headaches problems.

B3
C

Food sources of Vitamins

B3
Avocados, brewer's yeast, broccoli, carrots, cheese, corn flour, dates, eggs, figs, fish, kidney, liver, milk, meat (lean), peanuts (roasted), potatoes, poultry (white meat), prunes, tomatoes, wheat germ, whole wheat.

C
Berries, black currants, broccoli, brussels sprouts, cabbage, cantaloupe, cauliflower, cherry juice (acerola), citrus fruits, guava, horseradish, kiwi, peppers (red, green) potatoes, rose hips, spinach, strawberries, tomatoes, turnips, vegetables (green leafy) watercress.

Herb sources of Vitamins

B3
Alfalfa, burdock, dandelion, fenugreek, kelp, parsley, sage.

C
Alfalfa, burdock, boneset, catnip, capsicum, chickweed, dandelion, garlic, hawthorn, horseradish, kelp, parsley, plantain, papaya, rose hips, shepherd's purse, strawberry, watercress, yellow dock.

HEADACHES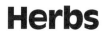

Herbs

These are the herbs that have been shown to help people suffering from headaches.

Feverfew	Mint	Ginko	Irish moss plant
Chamomile	Rosemary	Lavender	Burdock
Catnip	Sage	Valerian	Marjoram
Marshmallow	Thyme	Calendula	Cayenne

These are the herbs that have been shown to help people suffering from *migraine* headaches.

Feverfew	Lavender	Strawberry
Peppermint	Valerian	Blackberry
Nettle		

Food

These are the foods that have been shown to help people suffering from headaches.

Fish	Grains	Nuts
Fish oil	Whole grain bread	Seeds
Ginger	Vegetables	Dairy
Spinach	Raw salad	Eggs
Onion	Fruits	

HEADACHES

 Food

These are the foods that have been shown to aggravate headaches.

Chocolate	Nuts	Preservatives, MSG,
Caffeine	Ice cream	and Aspartame
Cured meats	Bread	Salt
Aged cheese	Cereal	

These are the foods have been shown to aggravate *migraine* headaches.

Dairy products	Eggs	Rye
Wheat	Oranges	Beets
Chocolate	Tomatoes	

Some people are affected by the following foods due to the lack of an enzyme that breaks down amines:

Avocados	Eggplant	Figs
Bananas	Pineapple	Onions
Cabbage	Potato	Peanut butter

HEADACHES

Home remedies

MAESTRO MUSIC PLEASE
* Soft music has a calming effect for migraine headaches.

ANOINT YOURSELF QUEEN
* On the forehead place a few drops of one of the essential oils: sage, rosemary, thyme, lavender. You can buy these oils at any health food store or even discount stores.

HEALING HANDS
* Massage the head and the back of the neck.

WHOLE BODY HEAL
* Place a towel or washcloth soaked in chamomile tea on back , shoulders and neck. Use this compress as hot as possible. If skin reddens, use St. John's wort oil on skin.

* Use a mustard plaster on your abdomen at the beginning of a headache. Mix 1 tablespoon of mustard powder with 3 tablespoons of flour. Add water to make paste. Place oil on skin before applying plaster.

HEADY IDEAS
* Hold a bag of ice on painful area for 15 minutes. Tie a headband around your head. It lessens the pounding of a migraine.

HEADACHES

Home remedies

SOMETHING TO SINK YOUR TEETH INTO
* In some cultures it is customary to chew on the barks of willow or black poplar trees to ease headaches.

VINEGAR VIGNETTE
* Soak a cloth with vinegar. Place on forehead, temples, and neck. The odor will scare the headache away.

* Boil equal parts of vinegar and warm water. Inhale the steam.

 A few more ideas

Headaches fall into two categories -- tension or vascular. Tension headaches result from involuntary contractions of the neck, scalp and forehead muscles. Stress, mostly occurring during election years, is a major cause. Vascular headaches, which include migraine, hunger or high-altitude headaches, occur due to dilation of the blood vessels.

Chapter
17

HEMORRHOIDS

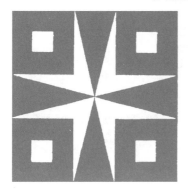

Don't take
this ailment
sitting down.

An herb with a history. Ginkgo is a useful herb for hemorrhoids. The ginko is the oldest living species of tree on the earth. The Chinese have been using the leaves for medicinal purposes for 4,000 years.

And for 4,000 years my Aunt Molly has kept an aloe vera plant in her kitchen. (I'm including all of the Aunt Mollys in our family tree.) She just loves this useful plant. The gel from the aloe vera plant can be discreetly placed so as to eliminate the pain and itching of hemorrhoids.

HEMORRHOIDS

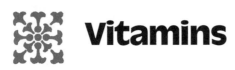 **Vitamins**

These are the vitamins that have been shown to help people suffering from hemorrhoids.

A	B12	E
Acidophilus*	Choline	Lecithin
B complex	Inositol	P
B6	C	

*This is found in supplement form or in active yogurt cultures.

Food sources of Vitamins

A
Carrots, dairy, fish liver oil, fruits (yellow), lemon grass, liver, milk, margarine, okra, vegetables (green, yellow).

B Complex
Apples, bananas, beans, beets, cabbage, carrots, cauliflower, corn, grapefruit, liver, mushrooms, onions, oranges, peas, peanuts, potatoes, spinach, turnips, watercress, yeast.

B6
Avocados, bananas, cantaloupe, chicken, eggs, liver, kid-

Herb sources of Vitamins

A
Alfalfa, burdock, capsicum, dandelion, garlic, kelp, marshmallow, papaya, parsley, raspberry, red clover, safflower, watercress, yellow dock.

B Complex
Kelp.

B6
Alfalfa.

HEMORRHOIDS

Food sources of Vitamins

Herb sources of Vitamins

ney, milk, nuts, oats, peanuts, peas, potatoes, soybeans, vegetables (green leafy), walnuts, wheat bran, wheat germ, yeast (brewer's).

B12
Beef, cheese, clams, cottage cheese, eggs, fish, lamb, liver, kidney, milk, oysters, sardines, tofu.

B12
Alfalfa, kelp.

B Factor: Choline
Brains, brewer's yeast, egg yolks, fish, heart, liver, peas, peanut butter, seeds, soybeans, turnip, vegetables, (green leafy), wheat germ.

B Factor: Inositol
Beans (dried lima), brains, cabbage, cantaloupe, grapefruit, heart, liver, molasses, oatmeal, oranges, peanuts, raisins, sesame seeds, soybeans, wheat germ, whole wheat bread, yeast.

C
Berries, black currants, broccoli, brussels sprouts, cabbage, cantaloupe, cauliflower, cherry juice (acerola), citrus fruits,

C
Alfalfa, burdock, boneset, catnip, capsicum, chickweed, dandelion, garlic, hawthorn, horseradish, kelp, parsley,

HEMORRHOIDS

Food sources of Vitamins

guava, horseradish, kiwi, peppers (red, green) potatoes, rose hips, spinach, strawberries, tomatoes, turnips, watercress, vegetables (green leafy).

E

Broccoli, brown rice, brussels sprouts, cereals (whole grain) corn, eggs, flour (enriched) kidney, liver, nuts, peas, soybeans, spinach, sweet potatoes, vegetables (green leafy), vegetable oils, wheat germ, whole wheat.

Lecithin

Corn, soybeans, vegetable oil, wheat germ oil.

P

Apricots, blackberries, black currants, buckwheat, cherries, citrus fruits (white skin and segment membranes), grapes, peppers (green), plums, prunes, rose hips, spinach.

Herb sources of Vitamins

plantain, papaya, rose hips, shepherd's purse, strawberry, watercress, yellow dock.

E

Alfalfa, dandelion, gotu kola, kelp, raspberry, rose hips, watercress.

P

Dandelion, rose hips.

HEMORRHOIDS

Herbs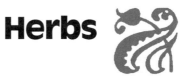

These are the herbs that have been shown to help people suffering from hemorrhoids.

Calendula	Ginger	Huckleberry
Yellow dock	Ginkgo	Echinacea
Bayberry	Mullein	Cayenne
Slippery elm	Marigold	Stone root
Witch hazel	Parsley	Aloe vera
Plantain		

Food

These are the foods that have been shown to help people suffering from hemorrhoids.

Apples	Pears	Blueberries
Beets	Whole grains	Blackberries
Broccoli	Bananas	Almonds
Carrots	Parsnips	Papaya
Cabbage	Plums	Pumpkin
Green beans	Prunes	Sweet potato
Oat bran	Yogurt	Winter squash
Lima beans	Cherries	

Juices {

Carrot	Celery	Lemon
Okra	Cucumber	Orange
Apple	Grapefruit	Pineapple
Beet		

HEMORRHOIDS
Food

These are the foods that have been shown to aggravate hemorrhoids.

Cracked grains in cereal or bread
Chocolate   Cola
Cocoa   Nuts
Coffee   Salt

 Home remedies

SIT ON IT
* To a cotton cloth add papaya juice and place on hemorrhoid area. Enough said.

SITZ BATH
* Add strong chamomile tea to a sitz bath.

BULK UP THAT DIET
* On a daily basis eat 1-3 tablespoons of unprocessed bran.

NATURAL OINTMENTS
* Use ointments made from Vitamins E, D, A.
* Also use ointment made from witch hazel.

CHILL OUT
* Place an ice pack on the area to reduce swelling. Never thought of placing ice there, did you?

Chapter

18

INDIGESTION

This ailment
is always hard
to stomach.

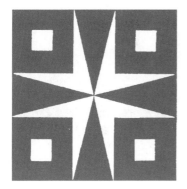

My father tries very hard to take to heart what his daughters believe in. When he had indigestion and I swore up and down on the healing power of chamomile tea, he figured the more cups he drank the better. I don't need to tell you how the poor man felt at the end of the day. Suffice it to say 3 cups per day is plenty.

It not always what you eat, but the conditions under which you eat. Relax, sit down and eat. And find pleasant eating companions.

INDIGESTION

 # Vitamins

These are the vitamins that have been shown to help people suffering from indigestion.

Acidophilus*	B3	B12
B complex	B5	Folic acid
	B6	

*This is found in supplement form or in active yogurt cultures.

Food sources of Vitamins

B Complex
Apples, bananas, beans, beets, cabbage, carrots, cauliflower, corn, grapefruit, liver, mushrooms, onions, oranges, peas, peanuts, potatoes, spinach, turnips, watercress, yeast.

B3
Avocados, broccoli, carrots, cheese, corn flour, dates, eggs, figs, fish, kidney, liver, milk, meat (lean), peanuts (roasted), potatoes, poultry (white meat), prunes, tomatoes.

B5
Beans, bran, brewer's yeast, chicken, eggs, fish (saltwater), kidney, liver, molasses, nuts,

Herb sources of Vitamins

B Complex
Kelp.

B3
Alfalfa, burdock, dandelion, fenugreek, kelp, parsley, sage.

INDIGESTION

Food sources of Vitamins

Herb sources of Vitamins

pork, potatoes, tomatoes, vegetables (green), wheat germ, whole grains.

B6
Avocados, bananas, brewer's yeast, cantaloupe, chicken, eggs, liver, kidney, milk, nuts, oats, peanuts, peas, potatoes, soybeans, vegetables (green leafy), walnuts, wheat bran, wheat germ.

B6
Alfalfa.

B12
Beef, cheese, clams, cottage cheese, eggs, fish, lamb, liver kidney, milk, oysters, sardines, tofu.

B12
Alfalfa, kelp.

B Factor: Folic Acid
Apricots, asparagus, avocados, beans, broccoli, carrots, cantaloupe, chick peas, egg yolks, flour (dark rye), liver, mushrooms, oranges, pumpkins, soybeans, spinach, sprouts, vegetables (green leafy), whole flour and wheat, yeast (tourtula), yogurt.

INDIGESTION

 ## Herbs

These are the herbs that have been shown to help people suffering from indigestion.

Chamomile	Slippery elm	Sage
Ginger	Alfalfa	Rosemary
Dandelion	Catnip	Thyme
Lemon balm	Fenugreek	Hops
Peppermint	Marshmallow	Anise
Cayenne	Garlic	Dill
Fennel	Parsley	Ginseng

 ## Food

These are the foods that have been shown to help people suffering from indigestion.

Garlic	Rice
Papaya	Cod liver oil
Bananas	Horseradish
Okra	Whole grains

Juices {

Blackberry	Coconut	Pear
Carrots	Cranberry	Spinach
Celery	Papaya	Tomato

These are the foods have been shown to aggravate indigestion.

Caffeine	Nuts
Citrus	Chocolate

INDIGESTION

Home remedies

A NEW FAVORITE-POTATO JUICE
* ✶ Grate potato. Using cheesecloth strain 1 tablespoon of juice. Combine with ½ cup warm water. Drink slowly.

TEA TIME
* ✶ ¼ teaspoon oregano and ½ teaspoon marjoram in 1 cup of hot water. Steep 10 minutes, strain and sip.
* ✶ 1 tablespoon of anise seeds in 1 cup of hot water. Strain. This acts as an antacid.
* ✶ ½ teaspoon of catnip or fennel in 1 cup of hot water. Steep 10 minutes, strain and sip.

COUSIN MITCHELL'S PRE-DINNER DRINK
* ✶ Try 2 teaspoon of apple cider vinegar in water. This helps digestion and also prevents food poisoning.

AUNT HANNAH'S FAVORITE
* ✶ Add ¼ teaspoon of cod liver oil to a glass of tomato juice. If you suffer from chronic indigestion drink before every meal.

THE RESTAURANT REMEDY
* ✶ Ever notice that at fancy restaurants they place slices of lemon in your water? Well they know that it helps aid digestion. Best results come from lemon in hot water.

CHEW THIS OVER
* ✶ Thoroughly chew a couple of sprigs of fresh parsley. All children will remember that Peter Rabbit went searching for parsley after he ate too many vegetables in Mr. McGregor's garden.

INDIGESTION
Home remedies

A NEUTRAL POSITION
∗ To neutralize stomach acid chew 1 teaspoon of rolled oats. (You can swallow after chewing.)

ABDOMEN PRESS
∗ Make a compress using chamomile tea. Do this by soaking a linen cloth with chamomile tea.

JUICE FROM ANOTHER PLANET
∗ How about green juice? Cabbage juice aids in digestion. Dilute a cupful of juice with water. Drink 1/2 cup, lukewarm 2 times daily.

 A few more ideas

Papaya is an effective digestion aid. It contains enzymes which help break down food. You can either eat a fresh piece of papaya before meals, or drink a juice made of crushed papaya pulp combined with orange juice.

Chapter
19

INFECTIONS

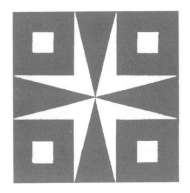

You can't see them,
you can't smell them,
but boy can you
feel them.

Mankind is constantly impressing itself with wondrous new solutions to all medical ailments. Well Mother Nature always has the last laugh. It seems that some bacteria have become resistant to antibiotics.

In comes garlic to the rescue. An extract from fresh garlic cloves has been proven to be effective against two very dangerous antibiotic-resistant strains -- staph and strep.

INFECTIONS

 # Vitamins

These are the vitamins that have been shown to help people suffering from infections.

A	C
Beta-carotene	E
B Complex	

Food sources of Vitamins

Herb sources of Vitamins

A
Carrots, dairy, fish liver oil, fruits (yellow), lemon grass, liver, milk, margarine, okra, vegetables (green, yellow).

A
Alfalfa, burdock, capsicum, dandelion, garlic, kelp, marshmallow, papaya, parsley, raspberry, red clover, safflower, watercress, yellow dock.

Beta-carotene
Apricots, broccoli, canteloupe, collard greens, kale, mango, papaya, peppers, pumpkin, peaches, romaine lettuce, spinach, squash, sweet potatoes, tropical fruit.

Beta-carotene
Bay leaves (crumbled), basil, marjoram, parsley, sage.

B Complex
Apples, bananas, beans, beets, cabbage, carrots, cauliflower, corn, grapefruit, liver, mushrooms, onions, oranges, peas,

B Complex
Kelp.

INFECTIONS

Food sources of Vitamins

peanuts, potatoes, spinach, turnips, watercress, yeast.

C

Berries, black currants, broccoli, brussels sprouts, cabbage, cantaloupe, cauliflower, cherry juice (acerola), citrus fruits, guava, horseradish, kiwi, peppers (red and green), potatoes, rose hips, spinach, strawberries, turnips, watercress, vegetables (green leafy).

E

Broccoli, brown rice, brussels sprouts, cereals (whole grain), corn, eggs, flour(enriched), kidney, liver, nuts, peas, soybeans, spinach, sweet potatoes, vegetables (green leafy), vegetables oils, wheat germ, whole wheat.

Herb sources of Vitamins

C

Alfalfa, burdock, boneset, catnip, capsicum, chickweed, dandelion, garlic, hawthorn, horseradish, kelp, parsley, plantain, papaya, rose hips, shepherd's purse, strawberry, watercress, yellow dock.

E

Alfalfa, dandelion, gotu kola, kelp, raspberry, rose hips, watercress.

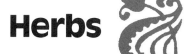

Herbs

These are the herbs that have been shown to help people suffering from infections.

Echinacea	Garlic	Cayenne
Hyssop	Goldenseal	Oregano
Calendula	Yarrow	

INFECTIONS

 ## Food

These are the foods that have been shown to help people suffering from infections.

Garlic	Figs
Yogurt	Pineapple
Shiitake mushrooms	Meat
Honey	Eggs
Blueberries	Milk
Cranberries	Bread
Raspberries	Yeast
Strawberries	Soy flour
Plums	Wheat germ
Peaches	

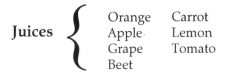

Juices {
Orange   Carrot
Apple   Lemon
Grape   Tomato
Beet

These are the foods that have been shown to aggravate infections.

Safflower oil	Fat
Soybean oil	Corn

INFECTIONS

Home remedies

IF YOU CAN STAND IT
* Eat 6 minced garlic cloves. If that's too hard, add the cloves to your salad or mix with butter and spread on toast.

HYDRO THERAPY
* To help the body throw off the infection you can use water. For hands, arms, feet and legs, soak them first in hot water and then in cold water. Three minutes in each temperature. Keep alternating until you have repeated the cycle three times. (Or until you get confused).

YOGURT, THE WONDER FOOD
* Yogurt with active cultures has the mineral acidophilus. Acidophilus can also be taken in tablet form. This is useful to take when antibiotics are prescribed. Antibiotics tend to reduce the natural acidophilus that is stored in your body.

BUILDING BLOCKS
* Block infections by keeping your immune system strong. Build your immune system with daily doses of vitamin C, garlic, tomatoes, broccoli and lots of fresh fruits and vegetables. The idea here is for the infections to pass you right by. You are no longer a weak target.

INFECTIONS

 A few more ideas

A fever associated with an infection is the body's way of fighting off the illness. Fever can even cause an infection to be less contagious. So you might want to give the fever a little time to fight the infection before intervening.

Best battle plan for infections. Repel them. A strong immune system wards off those invading infections. Suit up with proper nutrition, exercise and rest.

For a fungus infection you can make paste from brewer's yeast and vitamin E oil and apply to area twice daily.

Chapter
20

INSOMNIA

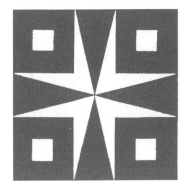

Put that time
to good use.
Earn another
degree.

My cousin Amy swears by an audio tape by Deepak Chopra called *Restful Sleep*. He has many ideas on how to create sleep. But the real treasure is his voice. So soothing and intelligent. Amy has yet to hear the entire tape as she keeps falling asleep in the middle of the tape. As a bonus her dreams are pleasant and she awakes to a general feeling of happiness.

Losing sleep deprives your body of precious time to rebuild and strengthen the very cells of your being.

INSOMNIA

 # Vitamins

These are the vitamins that have been shown to help people suffering from insomnia.

B Complex	B15	Folic acid
B3	Choline	C
B6		

Food sources of Vitamins

B Complex
Apples, bananas, beans, beets, cabbage, carrots, cauliflower, corn, grapefruit, liver, mushroom, onions, oranges, peas, peanuts, potatoes, spinach, turnips, watercress, yeast.

B3
Avocados, brewer's yeast, broccoli, carrots, cheese, corn flour, dates, eggs, figs, fish, kidney, liver, milk, meat (lean), peanuts (roasted), potatoes, poultry (white meat), prunes, tomatoes, wheat germ, whole wheat.

B6
Avocados, bananas, brewer's yeast, cantaloupe, chicken,

Herb sources of Vitamins

B Complex
Kelp.

B3
Alfalfa, burdock, dandelion, fenugreek, kelp, parsley, sage.

B6
Alfalfa.

INSOMNIA

Food sources of Vitamins

Herb sources of Vitamins

eggs, kidney, liver, milk, nuts, oats, peanuts, peas, potatoes, soybeans, vegetables (green leafy), walnuts, wheat bran, wheat germ.

B15
Apricot kernels, brewer's yeast, pumpkin seeds, rice (whole brown), sesame seeds, whole grains.

B Factor: Choline
Brains, egg yolks, fish, heart, liver, peas, peanut butter, seeds, soybeans, turnip, vegetables (green leafy), wheat germ, yeast.

B Factor: Folic Acid
Apricots, asparagus, avocados, beans, broccoli, carrots, cantaloupe, chick peas, egg yolks, flour (dark rye), liver, mushrooms, oranges, pumpkin, soybeans, spinach, sprouts, vegetables (green leafy), whole flour and wheat, yeast (tourtula), yogurt.

INSOMNIA

Food sources of Vitamins

C
Berries, black currants, broccoli, brussels sprouts, cabbage, cantaloupe, cauliflower, cherry juice (acerola), citrus fruits, guava, horseradish, kiwi, peppers (red, green), potatoes, rose hips, spinach, strawberries, turnips, vegetables (green leafy), watercress.

Herb sources of Vitamins

C
Alfalfa, burdock, boneset, catnip, capsicum, chickweed, dandelion, garlic, hawthorn, horseradish, kelp, parsley, plantain, papaya, rose hips, shepherd's purse, strawberry, watercress, yellow dock.

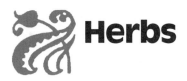 **Herbs**

These are the herbs that have been shown to help people suffering from insomnia.

Lemon balm	Hops	Ginger
Chamomile	Rosemary	Marjoram
Passion flower	Anise	Peppermint
Catnip	Basil	

INSOMNIA

Foods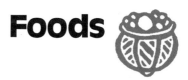

These are the foods that have been shown to help people suffering from insomnia.

Egg yolks   Brewer's yeast
Fruit   Peas
Cheese   Spinach
Poultry   Watermelon
Nuts

Juices { Apple Cherry Grape

These are the foods have been shown to aggravate insomnia.

Milk. It actually wakes you up!
No salt before bedtime.

Home remedies

STUFF IT
* A pillow stuffed with hops often brings sleep.

WARM MILK SUBSTITUTE
* Warm grapefruit juice.
* Add ½ teaspoon crushed nutmeg to hot water. Let steep 10 minutes and drink half an hour before going to bed.

INSOMNIA

Home remedies

IT'S ALL IN YOUR HEAD
* Apply ⅓ teaspoon crushed nutmeg oil to your forehead.

WASH AWAY YOUR WORRIES
* Take a lavender or rosemary bath. Immediately after the bath drink chamomile or ginger tea.

MOVE TILL YOU DROP
* In order to ensure a good night's sleep, the body must have adequate physical exercise. A guideline is 30 minutes a day prior to 4 PM. Or a short walk before bedtime.

AN APPLE A DAY
* Slowly eat an unpeeled apple before bed.

YOUR DAILY BREAD
* Don't like an apple a day? Try a piece of bread with butter and cayenne pepper. Remember to eat slowly.

UNCLE BEN'S METHOD: CHILL OUT
* An ice cold compress on the back of the neck.

THE QUEEN'S CUP OF TEA
* Of course one must have soothing tea to be properly relaxed. There are "Sleepytime" teas on the market which combine many of the herbs listed above.

BACKGROUND NOISE
* Background noise is soothing. You can buy a fancy "sleep machine," or play tapes of music, wind, rain, or waves. My Uncle Bernie has a better idea, he uses a fan that runs all night long.

Chapter
21

SINUS PROBLEMS

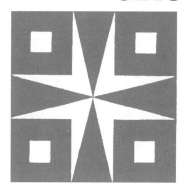

Compress, unclog,
chew and inhale.
Not an exercise
routine but methods
to relieve sinus
problems.

My friend Gina always seems to get a sinus problem every time I start talking about my career. Since the chances of stopping me from talking are the same as slowing down the earth's rotation, Gina has found a way to ward off her attack. She has an aspirin along with a strong cup of CAFFEINATED coffee. This way we are still friends.

Prevention is the key to avoiding sinus problems. The herb Echinacea is historically known as an infection fighter. The extract from the plant improves our immune system defenses. Taking either capsules, or tinctures (which are extracts made with alcohol) can prevent or lessen the duration of infections. Plus you can easily grow this in your herb garden.

SINUS PROBLEMS

 Vitamins

These are the vitamins that have been shown to help people suffering from sinus problems.

B Complex	C
B5	E
B6	P

Food sources of Vitamins

Herb sources of Vitamins

B Complex
Apples, bananas, beans, beets, cabbage, carrots, cauliflower, corn, grapefruit, liver, mushrooms, onions, oranges, peas, peanuts, potatoes, spinach, turnips, watercress, yeast.

B Complex
Kelp.

B5
Beans, bran, brewer's yeast, chicken, eggs, fish (saltwater), kidney, liver, molasses, nuts, pork, potatoes, tomatoes, vegetables (green), wheat germ, whole grains.

B6
Avocados, banana, brewer's yeast, cantaloupe, chicken, eggs, liver, kidney, milk, nuts, oats, peanuts, peas, potatoes,

B6
Alfalfa.

SINUS PROBLEMS

Food sources of Vitamins

soybeans, vegetables (green leafy), walnuts, wheat bran, wheat germ.

C
Berries, black currants, broccoli, brussels sprouts, cabbage, cantaloupe, cauliflower, cherry juice (acerola), citrus fruits, guava, horseradish, kiwi, peppers (red, green), potatoes, rose hips, spinach, strawberries, turnips, watercress, vegetables (green leafy).

E
Broccoli, brown rice, brussels sprouts, cereals (whole grain), corn, eggs, flour (enriched), kidney, liver, peas, soybeans, spinach, sweet potatotes, vegetables (green leafy), vegetable oils, wheat germ, whole wheat.

P
Apricots, blackberries, black currant, buckwheat, cherries, citrus fruits (white skin and segment membranes), grapes, peppers (green), plums, prunes, rose hips, spinach.

Herb sources of Vitamins

C
Alfalfa, burdock, boneset, catnip, capsicum, chickweed, dandelion, garlic, hawthorn, horseradish, kelp, parsley, plantain, papaya, rose hips, shepherd's purse, strawberry, watercress, yellow dock.

E
Alfalfa, dandelion, gotu kola, kelp, raspberry, rose hips, watercress.

P
Dandelion, rose hips.

SINUS PROBLEMS

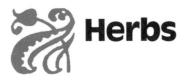 ## Herbs

These are the herbs that have been shown to help people suffering from sinus problems.

Sage   Slippery elm   Echinacea
Garlic   Ginger   Fenugreek
Goldenseal   Garlic   Red clover
Marshmallow   Horehound   Rose hips
Mullein

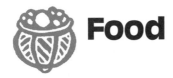 ## Food

These are the foods that have been shown to help people suffering from sinus problems.

Horseradish   Spinach juice
Raw fruit   Carrot juice
Raw vegetables   Hot liquids

These are the foods that have been shown to aggravate sinus problems.

Avoid dairy products but yogurt is all right.

SINUS PROBLEMS

Home remedies

UNCLOG THOSE PASSAGES
* Soak small strips of orange peels in apple cider vinegar.
  Let sit several hours. Drain. Add honey and cook
  until thick. At bedtime eat several strips. Great midnight
  snack!

COMPRESS
* Soak a linen cloth with ginger tea and place on forehead.
  Relieves congestion.

MAKE MINE STRONG
* Strong black coffee is said to do wonders.

CHEW ON IT
* Find a one inch square of honeycomb and chew on it for
  10 minutes. This can clear up congestion.

NOW YOU CAN INHALE
* Inhale the vapors from fresh ginkgo leaves that have just
  been boiled.
* Inhale salt water.
* Inhale the steam from chamomile tea.

ON THE ROCKS
* Take an ice pack and apply to the bridge of the nose and
  across the cheek bones. This will shrink inflamed tissues.

SINUS PROBLEMS
Home remedies

SWEET & SOUR
   * To a glass of water add 1 teaspoon of apple cider vinegar and 1 teaspoon of honey. Three times daily.

QUICK RELIEF
   * Take 1/2 teaspoon of horseradish and add a few drops of lemon juice. Do this both in the morning and the evening.

THE CEREBRAL MASSAGE
   * Combine 1 teaspoon of dry mustard with 2 tablespoons of vegetable oil. Massage this into your forehead.

GOOD NIGHT SWEET DREAMS
   * Place a bowl of sliced onions by your bedside at night. The fumes will chase away anything.

AN UNUSUAL INHALE
   * Quarter 1 large potato. Boil in 2 cups of water until tender. Remove the potato and inhale the steam.

THE EYES HAVE IT
   * 1 teaspoon of pekoe tea. Saturate cloth. Apply to eyes 4-5 times daily.

Chapter
22

SORE THROATS

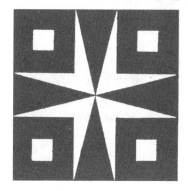

Inarticulate thoughts
that won't see
the light of day.

*Z*inc has long provided relief for sore throats. Studies have shown that zinc lozenges may prevent the cold virus from multiplying. They work quickly sometimes within 24 hours.

Sources of zinc are beef, chicken, oysters, crab, legumes, nuts, wheat germ, whole grains and milk.

SORE THROATS

 Vitamins

These are the vitamins that have been shown to help people suffering from sore throats.

A	C
Acidophilus*	P
Beta-carotene	

*This is found in supplement form or in active yogurt cultures.

Food sources of Vitamins

A
Carrots, dairy, fish, olive oil, fruits (yellow), lemon grass, liver, milk, margarine, okra, vegetables (green, yellow).

Beta-carotene
Apricots, broccoli, cantaloupe, collard greens, kale, mangoes, papayas, peppers, pumpkins, peaches, romaine lettuce, spinach, squash, sweet potatoes, tropical fruit.

C
Berries, black currants, broccoli, brussels sprouts, cabbage, cantaloupe, cauliflower, cherry juice (acerola), citrus fruits, guava, horseradish, kiwi, pep-

Herb sources of Vitamins

A
Alfalfa, burdock, capsicum, dandelion, garlic, kelp, marshmallow, papaya, parsley, raspberry, red clover, safflower, watercress, yellow dock.

Beta-carotene
Bay leaves (crumbled), basil, marjoram, parsley, sage.

C
Alfalfa, burdock, boneset, catnip, capsicum, chickweed, dandelion, garlic, hawthorn, horseradish, kelp, parsley, plantain, papaya, rose hips,

SORE THROATS

Food sources of Vitamins

Herb sources of Vitamins

pers (red, green), potatoes, rose hips, spinach, strawberries, turnips, watercress, vegetables (green leafy).

shepherd's purse, strawberry, watercress, yellow dock.

P
Apricots, blackberries, black currants, buckwheat, cherries, citrus fruits (white skin and segment membranes), grapes, peppers (green), plums, prunes, rose hips, spinach.

P
Dandelion, rose hips.

Herbs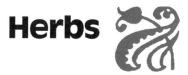

These are the herbs that have been shown to help people suffering from sore throats.

Plantain
Marshmallow
Slippery elm
Chamomile
Ginger
Yarrow

Garlic
Goldenseal
Hyssop
Myrrh
Echinacea

SORE THROATS

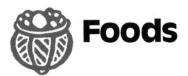 **Foods**

These are the foods that have been shown to help people suffering from sore throats.

Horseradish   Olive
Pineapple   Light diet
Vegetable broth

Juices { Grapefruit   Lemon
            Orange   Lime

These are the foods that have been shown to aggravate sore throats.

Limit intake of sugar.

In the case of laryngitis, avoid mint cough drops because they can dry out your vocal chords .

SORE THROATS

Home remedies

A STEAMY SCENE
- ✶ Inhale the steam from eucalyptus tea.

A GAGGLE OF GARGLES
- ✶ Sage tea
- ✶ Water with orange juice
- ✶ Water with 2 teaspoons of apple cider vinegar
- ✶ Saltwater
- ✶ Tea of your choice with honey
- ✶ Myrrh - 1 to 2 ml tincture in ½ cup of water

TAKE YOUR FOOT OUT OF YOUR MOUTH
- ✶ Politics aside, a hot footbath draws the blood away from the sore area.

TALK OF THE TEA
- ✶ Drink tea with honey and lemon juice. Mallow tea is especially helpful for laryngitis. Slippery elm bark tea coats the throat.

DO YOU BLOW HOT AND COLD
- ✶ You can use either a hot throat compress or a cold pack. Whatever mood you happen to be in.

ACT FAST
- ✶ At the beginning of a sore throat eat garlic cloves or onions. This should prevent laryngitis as no one will stay around you long enough to have a conversation.

SORE THROATS
Home remedies

TOSS HYGIENE OUT THE WINDOW
* Throw away your toothbrush. Germs gather there. Replace your toothbrush regularly to avoid reinfecting yourself.

DRINKS YOU WON'T FIND AT YOUR LOCAL CAFE
* 1 tablespoon freshly grated horseradish in 1 cup of water.
* 1 tablespoon ground cloves (stirred in warm water).
* 1 tablespoon of honey in 1 cup of water.
* Or combine milk, eggs, and honey and drink.

 A few more ideas

Two ideas for the use of a pomegranate in healing sore throats. Drink the juice of the pomegranate or boil the rind and gargle the liquid that is produced.

Gargle grapefruit juice.

The leaves and flower of the hyssop are used to treat sore throats.

Violet tea and American ginseng are helpful in treating sore throats.

Chapter
23

STRESS

Find a cave.
Go live there.

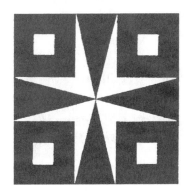

Learning how to relax and find your inner peace is the best way to cope with stress. My friend Emily is afraid of heights and could not go to a mountain top in India to find inner peace. Instead she uses an excellent audio tape by Belleruth Naperstak called *General Wellness*. (It's part of the *Health Journey Series* on audio tape.) Ms. Naperstak's soothing voice asks you to imagine and feel your most joyful place. This guided imagery is a great tool in learning how to calm your mind. Use daily for 10 minutes and you will feel the stress just melt away.

STRESS

 # Vitamins

These are the vitamins that have been shown to help people suffering from stress.

B Complex	B6	C
B2	B15	E
B5	Folic acid	Lecithin

Food sources of Vitamins

B Complex
Apples, bananas, beans, beets, cabbage, carrots, cauliflower, corn, grapefruit, liver, mushrooms, onions, oranges, peas, peanuts, potatoes, spinach, turnips, watercress, yeast.

B2
Avocados, beans, cheese, currants, eggs, fish, kidney, liver, milk, molasses, nuts, vegetables (green leafy), yeast.

B5
Beans, bran, brewer's yeast, chicken, eggs, fish (salt water), kidney, liver, molasses, nuts, pork, potatoes, tomatoes, vegetables (green), wheat germ, whole grains.

Herb sources of Vitamins

B Complex
Kelp.

STRESS

Food sources of Vitamins	*Herb sources of Vitamins*

B6
Avocado, bananas, brewer's yeast, cantaloupe, chicken, eggs, liver, kidney, milk, nuts, oats, peanuts, peas, potatoes, soybeans, vegetables (green leafy), walnuts, wheat bran, wheat germ.

B6
Alfalfa.

B15
Apricot kernels, brewer's yeast, pumpkin seeds, rice (whole brown), sesame seeds, whole grains.

B Factor: Folic Acid
Apricots, asparagus, avocados, beans, broccoli, carrots, cantaloupe, chick peas, egg yolks, flour (dark rye), liver, mushrooms, orange, pumpkin, soybeans, spinach sprouts, vegetables (green leafy), whole flour and wheat (tourtula), yogurt.

C
Berries, black currants, broccoli, brussels sprouts, cabbage, cantaloupe, cauliflower, cherry juice (acerola), citrus fruits, guava, horseradish, kiwi, peppers (red, green), potatoes, rose

C
Alfalfa, burdock, boneset, catnip, capsicum, chickweed, dandelion, garlic, hawthorn, horseradish, kelp, parsley,

STRESS

Food sources of Vitamins	Herb sources of Vitamins
hips, spinach, strawberries, tomatoes, turnips, watercress, vegetables (green leafy).	plantain, papaya, rose hips, shepherd's purse, strawberry, watercress, yellow dock.
E	**E**
Broccoli, brown rice, brussels sprouts, cereals (whole grain), corn, eggs, flour(enriched), kidney, liver, nuts, peas, soybeans, spinach, sweet potatoes, vegetables (green leafy), vegetable oils, wheat germ, whole wheat.	Alfalfa, dandelion, gotu kola, kelp, raspberry, rose hips, watercress.

Lecithin
Corn, soybeans, vegetable oil, wheat germ oil.

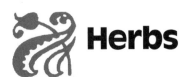 **Herbs**

These are the herbs that have been shown to help people suffering from stress.

Chamomile	Valerian root	Rosemary
Catnip	Hops	Sage
Peppermint	Ginseng	Basil
Passion flower	Lemon balm	Lavender

STRESS

Food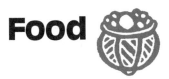

These are the foods that have been shown to help people suffering from stress.

Celery juice	Figs	Almonds	Apricots
Sesame seeds	Avocados	Sunflower seeds	Pumpkins
Oats	Mandarin	Beans	Lettuce
Wheat germ	Tangerines	Melons	Carrots
Tofu	Nuts	Peaches	
	Complex carbohydrates		

These are the foods have been shown to aggravate stress.

Alcohol	Cola
Caffeine	Fried foods
White sugar	Foods high in fat
Heavily spiced foods	

Home remedies

EXERCISE

* Experiment and find the best type of exercise for your body and schedule. And do it when you can; 10 minutes daily is enough to feel the effects. Don't feel you have to have a regimen in order to exercise.
* Exercise is the most efficient manner of dealing with stress. When exercising, your body produces endorphins which are the feel-good hormones you hear about. Endor-

STRESS
Home remedies

phines create a sense of calm ,wellness and happiness which washes away the stress you are experiencing.
* Chasing your spouse around the house to express an opinion is wonderful exercise.

WASH AWAY YOUR CARES
* Warm baths filled with herbs are very relaxing. Chamomile and lavender are the most common herbs. Some companies sell packages which combine stress relieving herbs.

MAESTRO, PLEASE
* If music soothes the savage beast it should help us humans. Studies have shown that classical music alleviates stress. Being from the Rock and Roll Hall of Fame city, Cleveland, very loud rock music works out the stress for my husband.

COUSIN SHAUN'S METHOD: TALK, TALK, TALK
* Sociability seems to lessen the stress we feel. My entire family will attest to the fun of listening to Shaun tell a story. Just by connecting with other people, we live happier, longer lives.

HUMOR
* As laughter can fight disease by exercising our internal organs, it can relieve stress by offering a positive, optimistic view of life.
* My grandfather Papa Lou loved a good laugh. He was always telling jokes and poking fun at life. Every Sunday for most our lives, my cousins and I would spend the day rolling on the floor with laughter at Papa Lou's stories. He lived to 85 and experienced good health

STRESS
Home remedies

and much happiness. He left to us a treasured legacy of laughter and joy. Not a day goes by that I don't hear his laughter in my mind.

A few more ideas

Since there is so much out there on the topic of stress - why we have it, what causes it, and what it does to your body - I won't repeat it here. What I will tell you is my method of dealing with stress. Maybe some of it will help you.

Four years ago I made a conscious decision to eliminate stress from my life.

First I evaluated all of my relationships; family, friends and job. I eliminated those relationships which brought me no joy. For those relationships that I couldn't eliminate, I readjusted my thinking. Only I could allow someone to cause me stress. I chose to ignore all stress producing comments or actions.

Next I made sure I stuck to my exercise program. Three times a week.

I take an hour each day and do something nice for my self (my soul).

I learned to meditate my own way. (See next page on meditation.)

Most importantly I keep a positive, optimistic attitude toward life.

STRESS
A few more ideas
Meditation

As your body needs to be properly aligned in order to enjoy good health, your mind also needs order. Once the body is fortified, the mind and spirit need nourishment. The mind needs to be clear of stress and tension. The spirit needs some room to surface.

I meditate.

This is a way to release stress and tension on a daily basis. I can also focus for a few minutes on issues outside of my particular life and let my spirit escape.

In keeping with adherence to simplicity, my method of mediation is easy. Having tried a few methods, most of which required my mind to become still - which is impossible for me - I found a technique that is used in yoga.

While I lie in bed, just before I want to fall asleep, I do the following. With my eyes closed, lying on my back with arms at my side, I take a body scan. Starting with my feet I imagine a white light of energy entering various body parts. Here is a brief example. The light starts in my left big toe, enters each toe individually, the foot, the arch, the calf and all the way up one side of my body over my head and back down. Next I focus the light on my internal organs. Afterwards I lie still and let both my body and mind experience a quiet state of relaxation.

Meditation is an effective way to prevent stress from settling in your body and causing illness.

Chapter

24

URINARY INFECTIONS

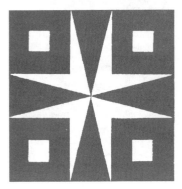

Not an ideal topic
of polite dinner
conversation.

But do spread the
word, for the
natural cures are
so easy.

In the back bedroom of my grandparent's house, Nanny (my grandmother) whispered to her daughters Gilda and Karen that cranberry juice would cure a urinary tract infection. It turns out that she was right. In 1991, Israeli scientists discovered that both cranberry and blueberry juice inhibit the bacteria which causes infections from clinging to the walls of the bladder.

URINARY INFECTIONS

 ## Vitamins

These are the vitamins that have been shown to help people suffering from urinary infections.

A	B6
Acidophilus*	E

*This is found in supplement form or in active yogurt cultures.

Food sources of Vitamins

A
Carrots, dairy, fish liver oil, fruits (yellow), lemon grass, liver, milk, margarine, okra, vegetables (green, yellow).

B6
Avocado, bananas, brewer's yeast, cantaloupe, chicken, eggs, liver, kidney, milk, nuts, oats, peanuts, peas, potatoes, soybeans, vegetables (green leafy), walnuts, wheat bran, wheat germ.

E
Broccoli, brown rice, brussels sprouts, cereals, (whole grain), corn, eggs, flour (enriched), kidney, liver, nuts, peas, soybeans, spinach, sweet potatoes, vegetables (green leafy), vegetable oils, wheat germ, whole wheat.

Herb sources of Vitamins

A
Alfalfa, burdock, capsicum, dandelion, garlic, kelp, marshmallow, papaya, parsley, raspberry, red clover, safflower, watercress, yellow dock.

B6
Alfalfa.

E
Alfalfa, dandelion, gotu kola, kelp, raspberry, rose hips, watercress.

URINARY INFECTIONS

Herbs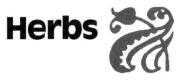

These are the herbs that have been shown to help people suffering from urinary infections.

Horsetail	Parsley	Rose hips
Chickweed	Cleaves	Dandelion
Nettles	Burdock	Goldenseal (if bleeding)
Echinacea	Marshmallow	Linseed oil

Food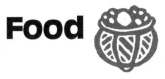

These are the foods that have been shown to help people suffering from urinary infections.

Cranberries	Blueberries	Parsley
Cranberry juice	Blueberry juice	Watermelon
Whey powder	Celery	Yogurt
Juniper berries		

These are the foods have been shown to aggravate urinary infections.

Citrus fruit	Carbonated beverages
Caffeine	Honey
Chocolate	

Don't take zinc or iron supplements until infection has healed.

URINARY INFECTIONS

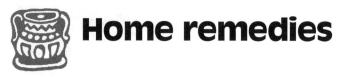 **Home remedies**

CRANBERRIES IT IS
* Cranberry juice is an old, old remedy.

WASH YOUR CARES AWAY
* Daily sitz baths. Add 1 cup of vinegar to the bath. Or add garlic juice or 2 cloves of crushed garlic to the bath.

DELIGHTFUL TEAS
* Parsley tea boiled in water 20 minutes does the trick.
* Drink 6-8 cups daily of any of the following teas: dandelion, stinging nettle, horsetail.

COOKWARE BEWARE
* Avoid aluminum cookware.

Chapter
25

WOMEN'S ISSUES

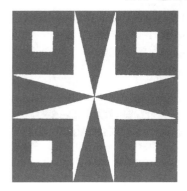

The original
feminist lives.
Mother Nature
provides
for her own.

M y cousin Deirdre is very spiritual. Back in college she decided to try yoga, feeling that it would condition both her body and mind. It worked. But she found an added benefit. It regulated her periods and decreased the pain from cramps. These internal workouts must have reset her internal clock and now her periods occur like, um . . . clockwork!

We'll start first with the Monthly Concerns; then the Nine-Month Concern.

WOMEN'S ISSUES

Menstruation Issues/PMS

Vitamins

These are the vitamins that have been shown to help women during menstruation.

B complex	B6
B 5	E

Food sources of Vitamins

B Complex
Apples, bananas, beans, beets, cabbage, carrots, cauliflower, corn, grapefruit, liver, mushrooms, onions, oranges, peas, peanuts, potatoes, spinach, turnips, watercress, yeast.

B5
Beans, bran, brewer's yeast, chicken, eggs, fish (saltwater) kidney, liver, molasses, nuts, pork, potatoes, tomatoes, vegetables (green), wheat germ, whole grains.

B6
Avocados, bananas, brewer's yeast, cantaloupe, chicken, eggs, kidneys, liver, milk, nuts,

Herb sources of Vitamins

B Complex
Kelp.

B6
Alfalfa.

WOMEN'S ISSUES
Menstruation Issues/PMS

Food sources of Vitamins

oats, peanuts, peas, potatoes, soybeans, vegetables (green leafy), walnuts, wheat bran, wheat germ.

E
Broccoli, brown rice, brussels sprouts, cereals, (whole grain), corn, eggs, flour (enriched), kidney, liver, nuts, peas, soybeans, spinach, sweet potatoes, vegetables (green leafy), vegetable oils, wheat germ, whole wheat.

Herb sources of Vitamins

E
Alfalfa, dandelion, gotu kola, kelp, raspberry, rose hips, watercress.

Herbs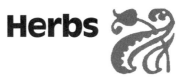

These are the herbs that have been shown to help women during menstruation.

Raspberry	Cayenne	Shepherd's purse
Nettle	Kelp	Peppermint
Feverfew	Chamomile	Yarrow
Dandelion	Lady's mantle	

Cramp bark (who named this?)

WOMEN'S ISSUES

Menstruation Issues/PMS

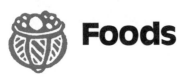 **Foods**

These are the foods that have been shown to help women during menstruation.

Fresh fruit	Lentils	Fish
Fresh vegetables	Nuts	Yogurt
Cereal	Sesame seeds	Kelp
Bread	Broiled chicken	Parsley
Beans	Turkey	Spinach
Peas		

These are the foods to avoid during menstruation.

Milk	Cabbage
Dairy products	Brussels sprouts
Red meat	Cauliflower
Fowl	Broccoli

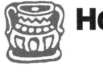 **Home remedies**

ADJUSTING THE FLOW
* Exercise, yoga.

TRY NOT TO HARM FAMILY MEMBERS
* Try a Calming Tea -Lemon balm, with a slice of fresh ginger.

WOMEN'S ISSUES
Menstruation Issues/PMS
Home remedies

TAKE A BITE OUT OF THE ORDEAL
* ✳ High protein snacks between meals: peanuts, sunflower seeds, sesame seeds, whole grain bread.

LORD GIVE ME STRENGTH
* ✳ Increase intake of calcium 10 days prior to period.

DON'T LET IT CRAMP YOUR STYLE
* ✳ For cramps take a Valerian tincture ½ teaspoon every half hour until pain stops.

Vitamins for PMS

These are the vitamins that have been shown to help women experiencing PMS.

C   E

Food sources of Vitamins

Herb sources of Vitamins

C
Berries, black currants, broccoli, brussels sprouts, cabbage, cantaloupe, cauliflower, cherry juice (acerola), citrus fruits, guava, horseradish, kiwi, peppers (red, green), potatoes, rose

C
Alfalfa, burdock, boneset, catnip, capsicum, chickweed, dandelion, garlic, hawthorn, horseradish, kelp, parsley, plantain, papaya, rose hips, shepherd's purse, strawberry,

WOMEN'S ISSUES

Menstruation Issues/PMS

Vitamins for PMS

Food sources of Vitamins

hips, spinach, strawberries, tomatoes, turnips, watercress vegetables (green leafy).

E
Broccoli, brown rice, brussels sprouts, cereals (whole grain) corn, eggs, flour(enriched) kidney, liver, nuts, peas, soybeans, spinach, sweet potatoes, vegetables (green leafy), vegetable oils, wheat germ, whole wheat.

Herb sources of Vitamins

watercress, yellow dock.

E
Alfalfa, dandelion, gotu kola, kelp, raspberry, rose hips.

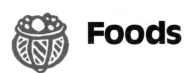 **Foods**

These are the foods that have been shown to help women experiencing PMS.

Eggs	Onions	Whole grains
Garlic	Beans	Fruit
	Vegetables	

These are the foods to avoid when experiencing PMS.

Milk	Fowl	Cauliflower
Dairy products	Cabbage	Broccoli
Red meat	Brussels sprouts	

WOMEN'S ISSUES

Pregnancy

The completed
work in
nine months.

HERBS GOOD FOR PREGNANCY
* Raspberry, ginger, alfalfa, nettle, dandelion, chamomile, blessed thistle, burdock, cramp bark, lemon balm, slippery elm.

HERBS TO AVOID WHEN PREGNANT
* Tansy, pennyroyal, goldenseal, angelica, motherwort, shepherd's purse.

FOLIC ACID
* Studies have shown that 400 milligrams daily of this vitamin B factor can prevent spina bifida and reduce the risk of neural tube defect by 50%. Sources include dried beans, liver, green leafy vegetables, orange and grapefruit juice.

Morning sickness

Vitamins

These are the vitamins that have been shown to help women suffering from morning sickness.

| B Complex | B6 |
| B1 | B12 |

WOMEN'S ISSUES
Morning sickness

Food sources of Vitamins	*Herb sources of Vitamins*
B Complex Apples, bananas, beans, beets, cabbage, carrots, cauliflower, corn, grapefruit, liver, mushrooms, onions, oranges, peas, peanuts, potatoes, spinach, turnip, watercress, yeast.	**B Complex** Kelp.
B1 Beans (dried), blackstrap molasses, bran, brewer's yeast, cereal grains (unrefined), egg yolks, milk, oatmeal, peanuts, peas, pork (lean) prunes, raisins, rice husks, vegetables, wheat germ, whole wheat.	**B1** Capsicum, dandelion, fenugreek, kelp, safflower, watercress.
B6 Avocados, bananas, brewer's yeast, cantaloupe, chicken, eggs, liver, kidney, milk, nuts, oats, peanuts, peas, potatoes, soybeans, vegetables (green leafy), walnuts, wheat bran, wheat germ.	**B6** Alfalfa.
B12 Beef, cheese, clams, cottage cheese, eggs, fish, lamb, liver, kidney, milk, oysters, sardines, tofu.	**B12** Alfalfa, kelp.

WOMEN'S ISSUES
Morning sickness

Herbs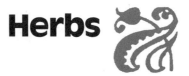

These are the herbs that have been shown to help women suffering from morning sickness.

Ginger
Raspberry
Peppermint

Foods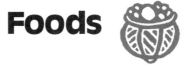

These are the foods that have been shown to help women suffering from morning sickness.

Oatmeal	Whole grains	Cabbage
Yogurt	Egg yolk	Organ meats
Wheat germ		

Home remedies

FIND GRANDMA'S HOT WATER BOTTLE
* With extreme nausea, place a hot water bottle on tummy for a *short* period of time.

FIND GRANDMA'S TEA POT
* Cup of ginger tea made from 1 -2 teaspoon fresh ginger.
* Peppermint tea - 1 teaspoon peppermint.

WOMEN'S ISSUES
Morning sickness

 A few more ideas

Morning sickness is that awful feeling when you reach for your maternity clothes. Most women complain of some type of morning sickness. The most powerful combatants are ginger pills. This is the same ingredient that you find in Chinese food, but it is compressed into a pill. I recommend 1-2 pills every 6 hours as needed.

Another easy method is a wrist band. Found at maternity stores or sometimes called sailor's bands, these bands put pressure on that point of the wrist that controls nausea. It works on the same principle as acupuncture.

Fatigue
 Vitamins

These are the vitamins that have been shown to help women suffering from fatigue.

B Complex.

WOMEN'S ISSUES
Fatigue

Food sources of Vitamins

B Complex

Apples, bananas, beans, beets, cabbage, carrots, cauliflower, corn, grapefruit, liver, mushrooms, onions, oranges, peas, peanuts, potatoes, spinach, turnips, watercress, yeast.

Herb sources of Vitamins

B Complex

Kelp.

Herbs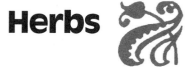

These are the herbs that have been shown to help women suffering from fatigue.

Alfalfa
Raspberry
Nettle

Foods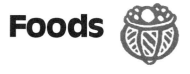

These are the foods that have been shown to help women suffering from fatigue.

Alfalfa	Beets
Egg yolk	Organ meats
Molasses	Dark green leafy vegetables

WOMEN'S ISSUES

Heartburn

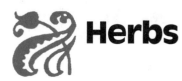

Herbs

These are the herbs that have been shown to help women suffering from heartburn.

Papaya   Anise
Marshmallow   Cumin
Slippery elm   Dill
Fennel

Food

These are the foods that have been shown to help women suffering from heartburn.

Milk
Yogurt
Papaya - fruit, tea, or in tablet form

These are the foods have been shown to aggravate heartburn.

Sugar
Cheese
Citrus fruit (except lemon and grapefruit)
Processed wheat

WOMEN'S ISSUES

Post Production Nursing

The knowledge my Aunt Molly possessed must have come down through the gene pool. She knew her stuff. To prevent soreness during nursing she advised use of mother's milk. Place it around the nipples. If the nipple becomes sore, use a wet tea bag. Not the decaffeinated tea since it is the tannin in the tea that works.

Vitamins

These are the vitamins that have been shown to help women during nursing.

B Complex
E

Food sources of Vitamins

B Complex
Apples, bananas, beans, beets, cabbage, carrots, cauliflower, corn, grapefruit, liver, mushrooms, onions, oranges, peas, peanuts, potatoes, spinach, turnips, watercress, yeast.

Herb sources of Vitamins

B Complex
Kelp.

WOMEN'S ISSUES

Nursing

Food sources of Vitamins	*Herb sources of Vitamins*

E
Broccoli, brown rice, brussels sprouts, cereals (whole grain), corn, eggs, flour (enriched) kidney, liver, nuts, peas, soybeans, spinach, sweet potatoes, vegetables (green leafy), vegetable oils, wheat germ, whole wheat.

E
Alfalfa, dandelion, gotu kola, kelp, raspberry, rose hips, watercress.

Lecithin
Corn, soybeans, vegetable oil, wheat germ oil.

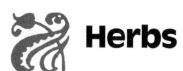 **Herbs**

These are the herbs that have been shown to help women during nursing.

Raspberry   Blessed thistle*   Alfalfa**
           Fenugreek*
           Marshmallow*
           Anise*
           Dill*
           Cumin*

Fennel - Seed boiled in barley water*

*Increases milk
**Makes milk richer (is this getting to sound like a recipe for a milk shake?)

WOMEN'S ISSUES

Nursing

Food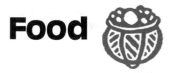

These are the foods that have been shown to help women during nursing.

Brewer's yeast*	Oats
Almonds	Honey

*Increases milk and energy.

Breast Infection

Vitamins

These are the vitamins that have been shown to help women during nursing.

A
E

C - At the first sign of infection take vitamin C. (You might need large doses so check with a knowledgeable health professional.)

WOMEN'S ISSUES
Breast Infection

Food sources of Vitamins

A

Carrots, dairy products, fish liver oil, fruits (yellow), lemon grass, liver, milk, margarine, okra, vegetables (green, yellow).

C

Berries, black currants, broccoli, brussels sprouts, cabbage, cantaloupe, cauliflower, cherry juice (acerola), citrus fruits, guava, horseradish, kiwi, peppers (red, green), potatoes, rose hips, spinach, strawberries, tomatoes, turnips, watercress, vegetables (green leafy).

E

Broccoli, brown rice, brussels sprouts, cereals (whole grain), corn, eggs, flour (enriched), kidney, liver, nuts, peas, soybeans, spinach, sweet potatoes, vegetables (green leafy), vegetable oils, wheat germ, whole wheat.

Herb sources of Vitamins

A

Alfalfa, burdock, capsicum, dandelion, garlic, kelp, marshmallow, papaya, parsley, raspberry, red clover, safflower, watercress, yellow dock.

C

Alfalfa, burdock, boneset, catnip, capsicum, chickweed, dandelion, garlic, hawthorn, horseradish, kelp, parsley, plantain, papaya, rose hips shepherd's purse, strawberry, watercress, yellow dock.

E

Alfalfa, dandelion, gotu kola, kelp, raspberry, rose hips, watercress.

WOMEN'S ISSUES
Breast Infection

Herbs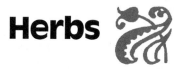

These are the herbs that have been shown to help women suffering from breast infections.

Echinacea	Parsley*
Dandelion	Sage*
Garlic	

*To dry up milk.

Food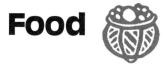

These are the foods that have been shown to help women suffering from breast infections.

Green tea
Brewer's yeast

Note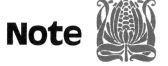

A thin layer of honey or almond oil will soothe cracked nipples.

WOMEN'S ISSUES

 ## A few more ideas

Raspberry tea is an especially good herb for women. It's effective for general health as well as specific pregnancy concerns. Studies have shown that drinking raspberry tea during the last trimester of pregnancy eases delivery.

During the last trimester of each of my pregnancies, I drank a cup a day of raspberry tea. I'm not saying that the tea has magical powers, but both of my deliveries were easy!

Table I

Herbs to use with caution

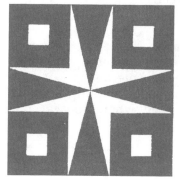

The power
of nature
must be
respected.

This is a table of herbs about which the experts disagree. Some consider these herbs dangerous, others will use them with caution. Generally, I do not include these herbs in this book. However, don't rule them out entirely when discussing your course of treatment with a knowledgeable health professional.

During pregnancy avoid:
    Aloe - In high doses causes vomiting. Don't take internally.
    Shepherd's Purse - Stimulates uterine contraction.
    Chamomile
    Myrrh   **Sage** - Avoid large doses
    Fennel   **Elder** - Don't use bark
    Goldenseal **Thyme** - Avoid large doses
    Ginseng

Table I

Herbs to use with caution

Herbs to avoid for a variety of reasons:

Aloe	Don't take internally; high doses can cause vomiting.
Cayenne	1) Seeds can be toxic. 2) Excessive consumption can lead to liver damage and gastroenteritis. 3) Don't leave on skin for prolonged periods. 4) Avoid touching eyes when using cayenne.
Coltsfoot	Causes liver damage.
Comfrey	Use is restricted in Australia, Germany, Canada, New Zealand. Avoid using on dirty wounds.
Elder	Don't take if condition would be worsened by further drying or fluid depletion.
Feverfew	Chewing fresh leaves can cause mouth ulcers in some people. Don't use if taking blood-thinning drugs.
Ginger	Avoid if you have a peptic ulcer.
Ginseng	Avoid other stimulants, tea, coffee and cola while taking ginseng
Goldenseal	Avoid if you have high blood pressure. Eating the fresh plant can cause ulceration of mucous membranes.

Table I

Herbs to use with caution

Hyssop	The essential oil can cause convulsions in high doses.
Licorice	Avoid if you have blood pressure. Avoid if taking digoxin based drugs. Avoid if rapid heartbeat occurs.
Mint	Avoid prolonged use an inhalant; it can irritate the mucous membranes. Don't give to babies. Give to young children for no longer than one week. If breast-feeding, can reduce milk flow
Pokeroot	TOXIC! Fresh plant is FATAL.
Sage	Not for those with epilepsy; can trigger seizure.
St. John's Wort	If taken internally, can cause dermatitis when skin is exposed to the sun.
Thyme	Dilute well. Can irritate mucous membranes.
Valerian	If taken for more than 2-3 weeks without a break, it can cause palpitations and headaches. Avoid if taking sleeping pills or drugs.
Yarrow	Prolonged use can increase skin's photosensitivity. In rare cases, can cause severe allergic rash.

Table I

Herbs to use with caution

 A few more ideas

U se common sense. Herbs are medicine. Tell your doctor, or other health professional, if and when you are using them. Herbs work on your body the same way that allopathic (western) medicines do. Therefore, you have to be careful which combinations are being used at the same time.

My friend used herbs while she was undergoing chemotherapy and her recovery was excellent. The two systems can work well together. But mixing the wrong combination of herbs and allopathic medicines could be dangerous.

Doctors are becoming more comfortable with holistic medicines so be sure to discuss any herbs you'd like to include in your treatment program.

Coordinate all treatments with your health professionals!

Table II
Food and herbal sources of vitamins

All you need to know about food and herbs sources of vitamins.

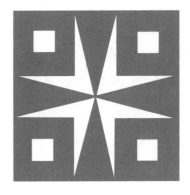

Food sources of Vitamins

A
Carrots, dairy products, fish liver oil, fruits (yellow), lemon grass, liver, milk, margarine, okra, vegetables (green and yellow).

Beta-carotene
Apricots, broccoli, cantaloupe, collard greens, kale, mangoes, papayas, peppers, pumpkins,

Herb sources of Vitamins

A
Alfalfa, burdock, capsicum, dandelion, garlic, kelp, marshmallow, papaya, parsley, raspberry, red clover, safflower, watercress, yellow dock.

Beta-carotene
Bay leaves (crumbled), basil, marjoram, parsley, sage.

Table II

Food sources of Vitamins	Herb sources of Vitamins
peaches, romaine lettuce, spinach, squash, sweet potatoes, tropical fruit.	
B Complex Apples, bananas, beans, beets, cabbage, carrots, cauliflower, corn, grapefruit, liver, mushrooms, onions, oranges, peas, peanuts, potatoes, spinach, turnips, watercress, yeast.	**B Complex** Kelp.
B1 (Thiamine) Beans (dried), blackstrap molasses, bran, brewer's yeast, cereal grains (unrefined), eggs yolks, milk, oatmeal, peanuts, peas, pork (lean) prunes, raisins, rice husks, vegetables, wheat germ, whole wheat.	**B1 (Thiamine)** Capsicum, dandelion, fenugreek, kelp, safflower, watercress.
B2 (Riboflavin) Avocados, beans, brewer's yeast, cheese, currants, eggs, fish, kidney, liver, milk, molasses, nuts, vegetables (green leafy).	
B3 (Niacin) Avocados, brewer's yeast, broccoli, carrots, cheese, corn flour, dates, eggs, figs, fish, kidney, liver, milk, meat (lean), pea-	**B3 (Niacin)** Alfalfa, burdock dandelion, fenugreek, kelp, parsley, sage.

Table II

Food sources of Vitamins	Herb sources of Vitamins

nuts (roasted), potatoes, poultry (white meat), prunes, tomatoes, wheat germ, whole wheat.

B5 (Pantothenic Acid)
Beans, bran, brewer's yeast, chicken, eggs, fish (saltwater), kidney, liver, molasses, nuts, pork, potatoes, tomatoes, vegetables (green), wheat germ, whole grains.

B6 (Pyridoxine)
Avocados, bananas, brewer's yeast, cantaloupe, chicken, eggs, liver, kidney, milk, nuts, oats, peanuts, peas, potatoes, soybeans, walnuts, wheat bran, vegetables (green leafy), wheat germ.

B6 (Pyridoxine)
Alfalfa.

B12 (Cobalamin)
Beef, cheese, clams, cottage cheese, eggs, fish, lamb, liver, kidney, milk, oysters, sardines, tofu.

B12 (Cobalamin)
Alfalfa, kelp.

B15 (Pangamic Acid)
Apricot kernels, brewer's yeast, brown rice (whole), pumpkin seeds, sesame seeds, whole grains.

Table II

Food sources of Vitamins	Herb sources of Vitamins

B17 (Laetrile)
Alfalfa seeds, almonds, apples, apricots, beans (broad), berries, buckwheat seeds, cherries, nectarines, papayas, peaches, plums.

B Factor: Choline
Brains, brewer's yeast, egg yolks, fish, heart, liver, peas, peanut butter, seeds, soybeans, turnips, vegetables (green leafy), wheat germ.

B Factor: Folic Acid
Apricots, asparagus, avocados, beans, broccoli carrots, canta-loupe, chick peas, egg yolks, flour (dark rye), liver, mush-rooms, oranges, pumpkin, soy-beans, spinach sprouts, veg-etables (green leafy), whole flour and wheat, yeast (tourtula), yogurt.

B Factor: Inositol
Beans (dried lima), brains, brewer's yeast, cabbage, canta-loupe, grapefruit, heart, liver, molasses, oatmeal, oranges, peanuts, raisins, sesame seed, soybeans, wheat germ, whole wheat bread.

Table II

Food sources of Vitamins	*Herb sources of Vitamins*
C Berries, black currants, broccoli, brussels sprouts, cabbage, cantaloupe, cauliflower, cherry juice (acerola), citrus fruits, guava, horseradish, kiwi, peppers (red and green), potatoes, rose hips, spinach, strawberries, tomatoes, turnips, watercress, vegetables (green leafy).	**C** Alfalfa, burdock, boneset, catnip, capsicum, chickweed, dandelion, garlic, hawthorn, horseradish, kelp, parsley, plantain, papaya, rose hips, shepherd's purse, strawberry, watercress, yellow dock.
D Dairy products, egg yolks, fish liver oils, herring, milk, salmon, spinach, tuna.	**D** Alfalfa, watercress.
E Broccoli, brown rice, brussels sprouts, cereals (whole grain), corn, eggs, flour(enriched) kidney, liver, nuts, peas, soybeans, spinach, sweet potatoes, vegetables (green leafy), vegetable oils, wheat germ, whole wheat.	**E** Alfalfa, dandelion, gotu kola, kelp, raspberry, rose hips, watercress.

F (Unsaturated Fatty Acids)
Almonds, avocados, black currant oil, cod liver oil, corn oil, cottonseed, flaxseed oil, linseed oil, peanuts, pecans, primrose oil, safflower oil, sunflower oil, soybean oil, wheat germ.

Table II

Food sources of Vitamins	Herb sources of Vitamins
G (Riboflavin) Green leafy vegetables.	**G (Riboflavin)** Alfalfa, capsicum, dandelion, gotu kola, kelp.
H (Biotin) Beef, bran, brewer's yeast, chicken, egg yolks, fish (saltwater), fruits, lamb, liver, kidney, milk, molasses, nuts, rice (unrefined), pork, sprouts, soy flour, wheat germ, vegetables (green leafy), molasses (blackstrap), safflower oil, soybean oil, sprouts, vegetables (green leafy, root).	
K (Menadione) Egg yolk, fish liver oils, legumes, liver, molasses (blackstrap), safflower oil, soy bean oil, sprouts, vegetables (green leafy, root).	**K (Menadione)** Alfalfa, kelp.
Lecithin Corn, soybeans, vegetable oil, wheat germ oil.	
P (Bioflavonoid) Apricots, blackberries, black currants, buckwheat, cherries, citrus fruits (white skin and segment membranes), grapes, peppers (green), plums, prunes, rose hips, spinach.	**P (Bioflavonoid)** Dandelion, rose hips.

Table II

Food sources of Vitamins	*Herb sources of Vitamins*

PABA
Bran, brewer's yeast, kidney, liver, molasses, rice, wheat germ, whole grains,.

T
Egg yolks, sesame seeds, tahini.

T
Plantain, alfalfa.

U
Cabbage (raw), celery juice (raw), sauerkraut.

U
Alfalfa.

Notes

* Steam, bake or stir fry vegetables to prevent loss of vitamins during cooking.

* Acidophilus is actually a bacteria although you will find its supplement form in the vitamin section. A food source is yogurt.

BIBLIOGRAPHY

Andrecht, Venus Catherine. *The Herb Lady's Notebook.* Ramona, CA: Ransom Hill Press, 1994.

Back, Phillippa. *The Illustrated Herbal.* New York: Crescent Books, 1987.

Buchman, Dian Dincin. *Dian Dincin Buchman's Herbal Medicine.* New York: Gramercy Publ. Co., 1979.

Cameron, Myra. *Treasury of Home Remedies.* Englewood Cliffs, N.J.: Prentice-Hall, 1987.

Carper, Jean. *Food, Your Miracle Medicine; How Food Can Prevent and Cure Over 100 Symptoms and Problems.* New York: Harper Collins, 1993.

Carse, Mary. *Herbs of the Earth: a self-teaching guide to healing remedies: using North American Plants.* Hinesburg, VT: Upper Access Publishers, 1989.

Hallowell, Michael. *Herbal Healing: a practical introduction to medicinal herbs.* Garden City Park, N.Y.: Avery Publishing Group, 1994

Leuog, Albert Y. *Chinese Herbal Remedies.* New York: Universe Books, 1984.

Lust, John B. Tierra, Michael. *The Natural Remedy Bible.* New York: Pocket Books, 1990.

Mabey, Richard. *The New Age Herbalist: How to use herbs for healing, nutrition, body care and relaxation.* New York: Macmillan Publ. Co., 1988.

Mindell, Earl. *Earl Mindell's Herb Bible.* New York: Fireside Pub., 1992.

Mindell, Earl. *Earl Mindell's Vitamin Bible.* New York: Warner Books, 1991.

Rodale's Illustrated Encyclopedia of Herbs. Emmaus, Pa.: Rodale Press, 1987.

Williams, Jude. *Jude's Herbal Home Remedies: Natural Health, beauty & home-care secrets.* St. Paul, Minn.: Llewellyn Pub., 1992.

Typesetting information

The body of this book is set in 11 point Padua. The head-lines are 24 point Antique Olive. Captions are 10 point Eterna.

About the author

Adrienne Selko writes a monthly column on holistic health for a nursing publication. She is the editor of *Business Quarterly* and is a partner in a public relations firm. A graduate of the University of Michigan with a degree in Business Administration, Adrienne has held positions in the field of consumer advocacy, including the Consumer Advocacy Division of the Illinois Attorney General's Office. Adrienne lives in Cleveland, Ohio, with her husband and two children.